LIVING WITH

VICTOR MARKS suffered ... holiday in Ireland, and had ... intensive care. He returned t... now working with Massey .... providing cardiac rehabilitation. He is also a member of the committee of the Wellington branch of the New Zealand Heart Foundation.

DR MONICA LEWIS is a general practitioner practising holistic medicine. Interested in well-being for the whole person, not just treating symptoms, she puts a strong emphasis on prevention of illness and reversal of disease to assist the body to achieve its healthiest possible state.

DR GERALD LEWIS, an invasive and clinical cardiologist with 30 years' experience in treating patients with heart disease, is deeply committed to rehabilitation and prevention. He has completed his doctorate on open heart surgery and its management, has been cited in *Who's Who in Medicine* for his work on high blood pressure, and was a foundation member of the Cardiac Rehabilitation Committee of the New Zealand Heart Foundation. He is currently setting up a cardiac prevention and recovery programme at SalusHealth in Auckland, New Zealand.

Overcoming Common Problems Series

For a full list of titles please contact
Sheldon Press, Marylebone Road, London NW1 4DU

The Assertiveness Workbook
A plan for busy women
JOANNA GUTMANN

Birth Over Thirty Five
SHEILA KITZINGER

Body Language
How to read others' thoughts by their gestures
ALLAN PEASE

Body Language in Relationships
DAVID COHEN

Cancer – A Family Affair
NEVILLE SHONE

Coping Successfully with Hayfever
DR ROBERT YOUNGSON

Coping Successfully with Migraine
SUE DYSON

Coping Successfully with Pain
NEVILLE SHONE

Coping Successfully with Your Irritable Bowel
ROSEMARY NICOL

Coping with Anxiety and Depression
SHIRLEY TRICKETT

Coping with Breast Cancer
DR EADIE HEYDERMAN

Coping with Bronchitis and Emphysema
DR TOM SMITH

Coping with Chronic Fatigue
TRUDIE CHALDER

Coping with Depression and Elation
DR PATRICK McKEON

Curing Arthritis Diet Book
MARGARET HILLS

Curing Arthritis – The Drug-Free Way
MARGARET HILLS

Depression
DR PAUL HAUCK

Divorce and Separation
Every woman's guide to a new life
ANGELA WILLANS

Everything Parents Should Know About Drugs
SARAH LAWSON

Good Stress Guide, The
MARY HARTLEY

Heart Attacks – Prevent and Survive
DR TOM SMITH

Helping Children Cope with Grief
ROSEMARY WELLS

How to Improve Your Confidence
DR KENNETH HAMBLY

How to Interview and Be Interviewed
MICHELE BROWN AND GYLES BRANDRETH

How to Keep Your Cholesterol in Check
DR ROBERT POVEY

How to Pass Your Driving Test
DONALD RIDLAND

How to Start a Conversation and Make Friends
DON GABOR

How to Write a Successful CV
JOANNA GUTMANN

Hysterectomy
SUZIE HAYMAN

The Irritable Bowel Diet Book
ROSEMARY NICOL

Overcoming Guilt
DR WINDY DRYDEN

The Parkinson's Disease Handbook
DR RICHARD GODWIN-AUSTEN

Talking About Anorexia
How to cope with life without starving
MAROUSHKA MONRO

Think Your Way to Happiness
DR WINDY DRYDEN AND JACK GORDON

Overcoming Common Problems

Living with Heart Disease

Victor Marks
Dr Monica Lewis
Dr Gerald Lewis

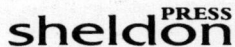

First published in Great Britain in 2003 by
Sheldon Press
1 Marylebone Road
London NW1 4DU

Original edition published in New Zealand in 2002 by
Tandem Press
2A Rugby Road
Birkenhead
Auckland
New Zealand

© Victor Marks, Dr Monica Lewis, Dr Gerald Lewis 2002

All rights reserved. No part of this book may be reproduced or transmitted in any form or by any means, electronic or mechanical, including photocopying, recording, or by any information storage and retrieval system, without permission in writing from the publisher.

British Library Cataloguing-in-Publication Data
A catalogue record for this book is available from the British Library

ISBN 0–85969–888–2

1 3 5 7 9 10 8 6 4 2

Typeset by Deltatype Ltd, Birkenhead, Wirral
Printed in Great Britain by Biddles Ltd
www.biddles.co.uk

Contents

Acknowledgements	viii
Introduction	ix
1 The heart and the things that can wrong	1
2 So who's at risk?	24
3 What the doctors can do	31
4 Beating the odds – recovery, rehabilitation and prevention	45
5 Living with heart disease	54
6 Body, mind and spirit	85
7 Dietary supplements	92
Appendix A: The drugs we take	95
Appendix B: Suggested reading	103
Appendix C: Useful addresses	106
Glossary	107
Index	109
At times of crisis	112

For Tanya, Bailey and Anne,
who were there when needed.

And to little Ella,
who we hope will benefit from our experience.

Acknowledgements

There are many people to thank for their help and advice in compiling this book, particularly the many members of Heart Support (Wellington), who unselfishly shared with us their own trials and tribulations of living with a heart condition. In particular, we would offer special thanks to Patsy and Evelyn, two women whose strength and courage have been an inspiration to us all.

We also acknowledge the support of the Williams family of Williams and Adam whose generosity has allowed the Wellington Heart Support group to flourish.

Thanks must also go to a number of learned individuals who gave their valuable time and generously shared their experiences and knowledge; hard-working GP and wonderful human being, Dr Jim Hefford; two magnificent lecturers at The Institute of Food Nutrition and Human Health, Massey University, New Zealand – Suzi Penny (BSc, MSc) and Jacques Rousseau (BA Honours); and for his meticulous editing skills, thank you Andrew Kellett.

These acknowledgements wouldn't be complete without offering our sincere thanks to all the doctors, consultants, surgeons, nurses and all those other wonderful people who have devoted their lives to looking after us when we are unwell. Thank you one and all.

Introduction

When someone is told that they're at risk of having, or already have, heart disease, they either turn a blind eye in denial, or they make an attempt to understand what is wrong and find out what they can do about it.

This book is for those who want to face the reality of their condition, get to understand it and take control of their own health.

Written with the practised understanding of a doctor, the expert knowledge of a heart specialist and the first-hand experience of a once ignorant patient, the book explains in simple everyday language the why? what? where? when? and how? of heart disease. Seen through the eyes of a layman, it's a straightforward common-sense view of what is now the number one killer in the Western world.

Heart statistics – the reality

Heart disease is the leading cause of death in the UK.

- Every two minutes someone in the UK has a heart attack.
- In the year 2000, 120,000 women died from a heart attack.
- To put this in perspective, over the same period 50,000 *fewer* women died from all cancers.
- One in three people who die of heart disease will be under 70 years of age.
- For 30 per cent of those who die from heart disease the first symptom will be their own sudden death.
- If you smoke you at least double your risk of having heart disease.
- Half of all continuing smokers will die early – on average 14 years early.

The encouraging fact is that heart disease is preventable and it only takes one small change to make a difference.

Statistics courtesy of The National Heart Foundation of New Zealand and the British Heart Foundation.

INTRODUCTION

What this book is about

> Prevention is better than cure.
> Thomas Love Peacock, *Melincourt* (1817)

Some facts and figures

Look at facts and figures on page ix. Frightening aren't they! And every year the figures get worse!

In the past, the great killers of our populations were the infectious diseases – tuberculosis, pneumonia, smallpox. But now, at the dawn of the twenty-first century, with these diseases having been mostly conquered, it is heart disease that is the great killer.

And it's not only the western world that is experiencing such high rates of heart disease. Increases are being felt throughout the whole world. In India, for example, a country in which heart disease was relatively unknown until recently, it is now estimated that within the next ten years it will become their number one killer.

However, there's an awful lot that we can do to reduce this terrible premature waste of human life, the causes of which so many of us either don't know about or are simply ignoring.

It is now well proven that heart disease is not only preventable but can also, if caught early enough, be held in check and in many cases even reversed.

(It's interesting to note that the same measures that prevent heart disease will also help protect us from cancer, Alzheimer's, arthritis, diabetes and most other degenerative disorders.)

Some more facts and figures

- Drug treatment to dissolve clots causing heart attacks (thrombolysis) has become routine in hospital coronary care units.
- Trials have shown that some groups of drugs (see Appendix A, The drugs we take) can reduce the incidence of heart disease by 30 per cent.
- The number of coronary bypass surgery operations has more than doubled, making it the most commonly performed operation of any kind.
- Coronary angioplasty (see p. 38) was first performed in America in 1978 and by 1991 more than 300,000 procedures were being

INTRODUCTION

performed each year. Ten years later these numbers have more than doubled.

Yet despite all our modern equipment and techniques, half of all heart attacks are still fatal. Most of those who die do so before they get to hospital and so never get the benefit of our modern technology.

So what can we do about it? Let's first look at what future technology is likely to offer us.

- New drugs will be perfected that will encourage new arteries to develop (collaterals) and bypass those that are blocked.
- New methods of investigation – CT calcium scoring, CT and MRI angiography – will be able to identify early indications of developing heart disease.
- New impregnated angioplasty stents and improved invasive surgical procedures will reduce the instances of possible complications.

But no matter what improvements there are in technology, the best weapon to fight this disease lies in our own hands – prevention (see Prevention, p. 49). It is our hope that while there will surely be many new procedures and drugs to help us combat heart disease, more and more people will become aware of the hugely important role that they themselves can play in fighting off this killer disease. You'll be surprised at just how much a few changes to your lifestyle will actually achieve in very real terms.

And that's what this book is about – to help you understand and make those changes. Many people, when confronted with the thought of making changes in their lifestyle, immediately throw up their hands, thinking that the changes they will be asked to make will disrupt their lives and life will never be as good again. How very wrong they are!

So before you delve too deeply into the book, let's have a quick look at what prevention is. It's about:

- Having regular checks to confirm that your cholesterol, blood pressure and glucose levels are in the ideal range. (See Chapter 3.)
- If you have a family history of heart disease, considering having a non-invasive heart check – coronary calcium scoring or exercise ECG test – at the age of 45 for men and 50 for women. If the

INTRODUCTION

results are negative, the tests should be repeated ten years later. (See Chapter 2.)
- Starting to take care of yourself and your heart as early as possible – heart disease, though it doesn't show itself until later, begins early in life – in our teens and twenties. (See Chapter 4.)
- Watching your weight, and for goodness sake not smoking! (See Risk factors you can change, p. 25.)
- A healthy diet is important and can be more enjoyable than you may think. (See We are what we eat, p. 54.)
- There is excellent evidence that in addition to a good diet, some dietary supplements can be beneficial to you. (See Chapter 7.)
- Regularly exercising – 30 minutes a day is all your heart asks. (See Keeping the body moving, p. 70.)
- Learning to keep stress to a minimum – we need some but most of us put far too much on ourselves. (See Coping with stress, p. 85.)
- There are many drugs available should you need them – but don't be like many people and assume that just because you're taking a particular drug you can ignore the other preventative measures you should be taking. (See Medication, p. 37.)

Now that doesn't seem too strenuous or unpleasant, does it? Of course there's more to it than just these brief headings – but this is exactly what this book is about. Through understanding your heart and how it works within your body, we'll show you how easy it is to adopt a lifestyle that will give you a long and fulfilling life.

The foundations for a healthy heart are laid down in our childhood and it is not uncommon to find the beginnings of the disease in teens and 20-year-olds. So if we start on this road to health with our children while they are still young, what a wonderful legacy we will be giving them and their own children.

1
The heart and the things that can go wrong

> All the knowledge I possess everyone else
> can acquire, but my heart is all my own.
> Goethe, *The Sorrows of Young Werther* (1772)

What our heart does for us

The role of the heart

The heart is a small pump, about the size of a man's clenched fist, located – not, as commonly thought, on the left side of our chest – but sitting comfortably right in the centre under the protective sternum and rib cage. Its job is to circulate our blood – which carries the oxygen and nutrients we need – around our body in a series of pipes called arteries, capillaries and veins.

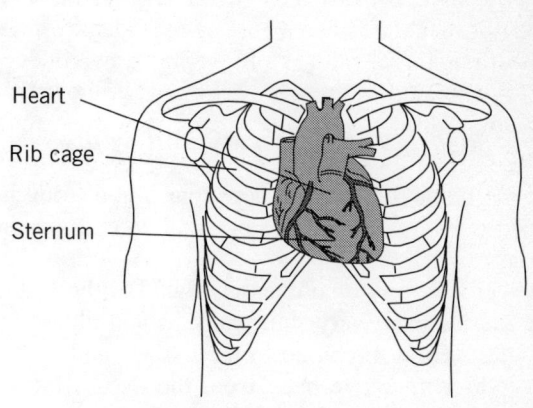

During an average 24-hour day this little pump will move enough blood to fill an average petrol tanker.

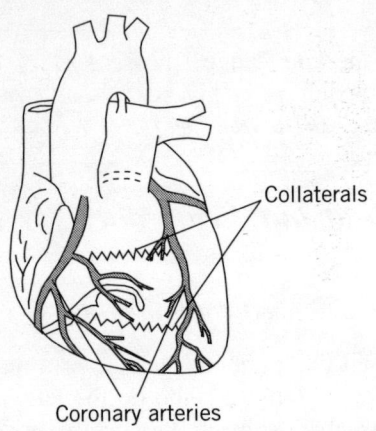
Collaterals
Coronary arteries

The heart gets its own nutrient supply through the coronary arteries, with oxygen-rich blood feeding into its own muscle (the myocardium). Overlapping these arteries is a secondary network of minuscule blood vessels called collaterals. These are our body's 'back-up': when the coronary arteries become blocked, the collaterals can enlarge and begin to feed blood beyond the point of the blockage.

Arteries, capillaries and veins

Arteries are the blood vessels that carry our blood from the heart to the tissues of the body. The arteries branch into ever-smaller vessels called capillaries.

Capillaries are the tiny blood vessels found at the end of the fine arteries. Capillaries have very thin walls, which allow oxygen and nutrients to move from the blood to the tissues, and carbon dioxide and waste products to move back from the tissues into the blood. The capillaries in turn connect to the veins.

Veins are the vessels that carry our blood back to our heart.

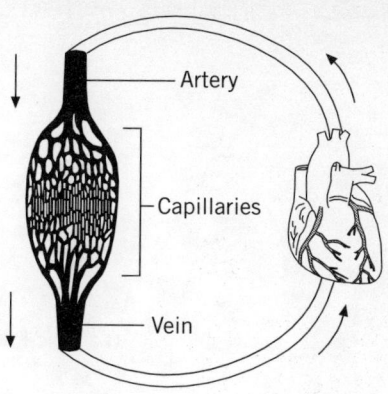

Blood pressure

For our blood to flow through our bodies it needs to be under pressure. When blood pressure is too high the heart has to work harder than necessary and that puts a strain on the heart muscle. High pressure can also damage the inside of the arteries, leading to heart attack, stroke or kidney failure.

About a quarter of the population has blood pressure that is greater than it should be; this condition is called hypertension and is often referred to as 'the silent killer' because most people don't realize they have it until they suffer a heart attack or a stroke. (See Hypertension, p. 9.)

Blood pressure readings

Because the heart pumps and then relaxes, blood pressure rises and falls. The higher pressure – the first number – called the 'systolic' pressure, should ideally read around 120 or less; the second number – the 'diastolic', should read around or under 80. If this were the case it would be shown as 120/80.

If blood pressure consistently reads above 120/80 you are moving into the realm of hypertension. Any reading over 140/90 may need further diagnostic tests. It should be noted that blood pressure readings increase as we get older.

Since blood pressure varies throughout the day the reading should be taken at a time when you are at rest and, ideally, for comparative reasons, at the same time each day.

In most cases medication can be prescribed to control high blood pressure. (See Appendix A – The drugs we take, p. 95.)

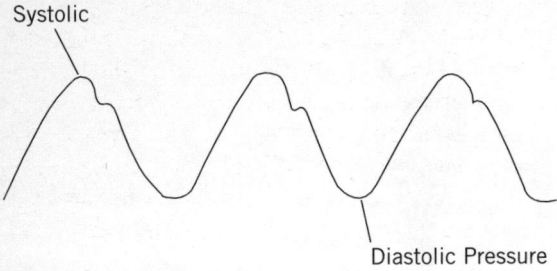

Men's hearts – women's hearts

As women are generally of smaller build than men, it makes sense that their hearts are also smaller and lighter, with heart rates that tend to be faster than those of their male counterparts.

A popular myth has it that women are immune from heart disease until after the menopause – but that is just what it is – a myth. Yes, a woman's chance of heart disease increases after menopause, but many show early signs and have heart attacks in their thirties and forties.

The symptoms of heart disease in women are similar to those in men, but women are more likely to describe a burning sensation in their chest and upper abdomen, rather than the heavy weight felt by males. These symptoms are frequently confused with indigestion and heartburn, and because stress testing in women is much less accurate than in men, angina in women is far harder to diagnose.

The things that can go wrong

> We are adhering to life now with our last muscle – the heart.
> Djuna Barnes, *Nightwood* (1937)

Heart disease

Heart disease (also referred to as cardiovascular disease) is the overall name given to the many various conditions that adversely affect the heart.

THE HEART AND THE THINGS THAT CAN GO WRONG
Coronary artery disease (CAD)

This is also referred to as either:

Ischaemic heart disease – from ischaemia – meaning lack of blood. In the heart this is usually due to:

Atherosclerosis – the process whereby the arteries become hardened and blocked. It is sometimes also called arteriosclerosis.

A health problem of our times, coronary artery disease is the name we give to the condition where the coronary arteries that feed the heart's muscles become blocked and thus starve the muscles of much-needed oxygen. It is a progressive disease that can build quite slowly and often remains undetected for many years.

Plaque

As fat builds up in the artery wall it attracts calcium and fibrous tissue, forming what is called plaque. Evidence of this can remain hidden for many years and only become noticeable when the build-up of plaque becomes large enough to reduce the flow of blood through the artery.

Although you are unaware of it, coronary artery disease usually starts in young adulthood and slowly develops undetected over the years to give its first indications later in life, when the narrowing slows the blood flow. These indications are usually noticed as chest pain when the body experiences exertion (see Symptoms, below) and can in some cases lead to a heart attack. (See Heart attack, p. 18.)

Why our arteries should become blocked is a complicated issue. The main causes (risk factors) include:

- family history (see So who's at risk? p. 24)
- lack of physical exercise (see The 'couch potato' syndrome, p. 28)
- smoking (see p. 28)
- bad eating habits (see p. 25)
- high cholesterol (see p. 25)
- high blood pressure (see p. 27)
- stress (see p. 28).

The good news is that, once detected, heart disease can be contained, and, in many cases, reversed.

THE HEART AND THE THINGS THAT CAN GO WRONG

Early detection

The earlier coronary artery disease is identified the easier it is to control. Don't wait for the symptoms to appear; ask yourself if any of the factors above apply to you, and if you answer 'yes' to more than one we strongly suggest you talk to your doctor. (See What the doctors can do, p. 31.)

Symptoms

For most people, the first sign that all is not as it should be is when they are doing some physical activity – mowing the lawn, running to get out of the rain or just playing with the grandchildren – and they feel an unusual pain across their chest. This can be a sensation of heaviness, a tightness or a feeling of pressure that may radiate to the neck and throat and in many cases spread up to the left shoulder and arm.

If you do feel such a pain when you exert yourself, the chances are that it's your heart telling you that not enough oxygen-rich blood is getting through to feed the heart muscle; it is being pushed just that little bit more than normal. What you could be experiencing is angina.

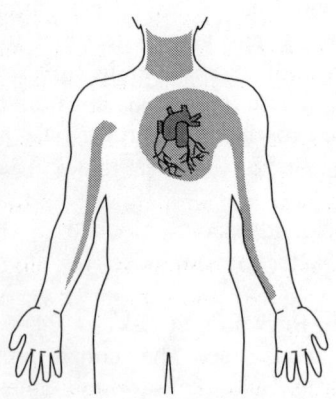

Unstable angina

If you feel these same symptoms while you are at rest, this could be more serious and indicate that there is indeed a growing blockage. It could be what's called *unstable angina* and you should see your doctor as soon as possible.

> **Angina pectoris**
>
> This is the medical name for the pain or discomfort you feel when there is insufficient blood getting through to the heart muscle. It's a warning that all is not well.
>
> It is generally felt when you physically exert yourself or you put yourself under emotional stress. You are also likely to experience it more after a meal or in the winter when you breathe in the cold air.
>
> If, on resting, the pain continues and is not relieved by medication, it could be the sign of an impending heart attack and you should immediately call an ambulance. (See What to do if you think you're having a heart attack, p. 19.)
>
> Angina can be relieved with medication, in the form of either a nitroglycerine spray or tablets. (See Appendix A, The drugs we take, p. 95.)

Treatment

The first line of attack on coronary artery disease is a change of lifestyle. Research throughout the world has shown that adopting an active, healthy lifestyle can not only hold the disease in check, but will in many cases actually reverse it. (See Beating the odds, p. 45.)

As well as modifying your lifestyle, you can take drugs that will help you combat and beat coronary artery disease. These are:

- *Beta-blockers*   These are used to lower heart rate and blood pressure, thus reducing the work the heart has to do.
- *Calcium-channel blockers*   Similar to beta-blockers, some can also open the arteries a little.
- *Vasodilators (nitrates)*   These improve the blood flow by causing blood vessels to relax and allow more oxygen and nutrients to reach the heart muscle.

For a full list of drugs and their brand names please refer to Appendix A – The drugs we take, p. 95.

Heart failure

The term heart failure is unfortunate as it's not that the heart has failed; it is just not working as well as it should. This is usually due to disease affecting either the heart muscle or its valves and could be caused by any one of the following:

THE HEART AND THE THINGS THAT CAN GO WRONG

- a previous heart attack (see p. 18)
- coronary artery disease (see p. 5)
- high blood pressure (hypertension) (see p. 9)
- valve disease (see p. 15)
- congenital heart disease (see p. 11)
- cardiomyopathy (see p. 10)
- myocarditis (see p. 10).

If it is diagnosed early enough, the workload on the heart can be eased with medication and you should be able to go on to lead a full and active life.

Congestive heart failure

This is the term given to the condition when there is excess build-up of fluid in the body. When the heart is not pumping with its normal force, blood returning to the heart can back up and become congested in the veins and tissues.

If the weakness is on the right side of the heart there will be swelling in the abdomen and lower legs and ankles.

If the weakness is on the left side, fluid can collect in the lungs, causing difficulties with breathing. This condition is called *pulmonary oedema*.

Symptoms

In the early stages of heart failure there may be no significant symptoms, although as time passes certain problems will arise. These fall into two categories:

- When the heart starts having difficulty pumping sufficient blood around the body, the body will react with feelings of tiredness, weakness and a general sense of feeling unwell.
- The other set of symptoms are a result of fluid congestion in the tissues. These show themselves as breathlessness, a cough and swellings of the feet, ankles, legs or stomach.

Treatment

Being diagnosed with heart failure will first and foremost mean a change in lifestyle where a balance must be achieved between resting and yet giving the body sufficient exercise to keep it working as efficiently as possible. It is also important to reduce the salt in

THE HEART AND THE THINGS THAT CAN GO WRONG

your diet, and not drink too much alcohol. (See We are what we eat, p. 54.)

Medicines will also play an important role in treatment, with doctors prescribing a combination of different medications. Among these are:

- *ACE (angiotensin-converting enzyme) inhibitors* These help to control symptoms and slow the advance of the disease.
- *Digitalis (digoxin)* This has been around for hundreds of years. Made from the foxglove, it slows the heartbeat and improves the circulation.
- *Diuretics* These help the kidneys rid the body of excess fluid and sodium.

Warning signs of heart failure

- shortness of breath
- feeling weak and listless
- swelling around the ankles and legs
- cough
- loss of appetite
- unusual weight gain

For a full list of drugs and their brand names please refer to Appendix A – The drugs we take, p. 95.

Hypertension

This is the technical name for high blood pressure. Although it might not sound particularly worrying, raised blood pressure causes an increase in the heart's workload and can eventually contribute to heart disease and other cardiac problems. High blood pressure can also damage the artery walls, leading to hardening of the arteries. (See Blood pressure, p. 3.)

Factors that contribute to hypertension include heredity, high salt intake, being overweight, tobacco smoking, high alcohol consumption, and physical inactivity. (See So who's at risk?, p. 24.)

Nowadays high blood pressure can be controlled by medication. (See Appendix A – The drugs we take, p. 95.)

At least one third of people who have a heart attack or a stroke have high blood pressure. High blood pressure has no symptoms, which is why it's often referred to as 'the silent killer'.

THE HEART AND THE THINGS THAT CAN GO WRONG

Aneurysm

An aneurysm is the name given to the condition where there is an abnormal bulge in a weakened blood vessel wall. It may occur as a result of artery disease, hypertension, a congenital abnormality or a tear in the blood vessel.

Early diagnosis of an aneurysm is vital as a delay may mean rupture. Minor aneurysms may be monitored with the use of antihypertensive drugs, although if they increase significantly in size then surgery may be required.

Cardiomyopathy

This is a condition where the heart muscle (myocardium) deteriorates and is unable to pump blood with the required force. It has a number of causes, including viral diseases and excess alcohol intake. There are a number of other rare causes, although most cases of cardiomyopathy are called 'idiopathic' – meaning 'the cause is unknown'.

Treatment for cardiomyopathy is generally the same as the treatment for heart failure.

Myocarditis

This refers to inflammation of the heart muscle, generally caused by viral, bacterial or fungal infection, toxic drug poisoning, or diseases such as rheumatic fever, diphtheria, or tuberculosis. Symptoms of myocarditis include fever, mild chest pains, aching joints and an abnormally rapid heartbeat.

Arterial embolism

Occasionally, as plaque builds up on an artery wall, a small part can become dislodged and be carried through the circulatory system to become lodged somewhere else. Such a loose piece of plaque or clot is called an embolus. When an artery is blocked by an embolus it is called an arterial embolism.

Early detection of an embolism is very important because, depending on where the blockage is, it can be the cause of a heart attack or stroke. If an embolism is suspected your doctor may ask you to have either an angiogram (see Angiography, p. 35) or an ultrasound test (see Echocardiography, p. 35).

THE HEART AND THE THINGS THAT CAN GO WRONG

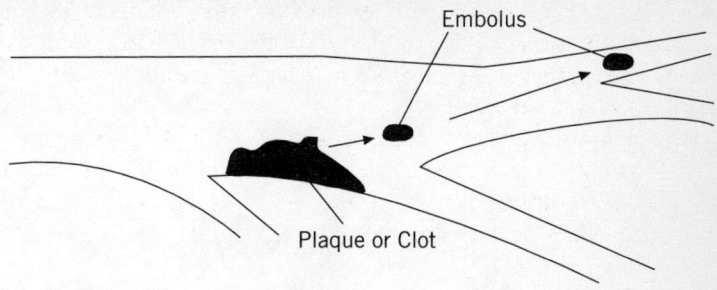

Treatment for an embolism is usually medication – a blood clot-dissolving agent.

Congenital heart disease

Congenital heart disease is the name given to heart disorders that are present when we are born. These conditions can be diagnosed before birth, immediately after birth or during childhood. Sometimes the condition is so minor that the symptoms don't show themselves until adolescence or adulthood.

What causes congenital heart disease?

If your child is born with a congenital heart disorder your first reaction will most probably be to ask, 'Why me?', 'What went wrong?' or 'Is it my fault?' The answer to the first two questions is simply – we don't know; and the answer to the last is – certainly not! It's not a hereditary disease and there is no evidence to show that it is anything other than a matter of chance.

Classification of congenital defects

Common defects include:

- abnormal blood vessels that restrict the flow of blood
- faulty valves that either restrict or block blood flow
- incorrect connections between heart, arteries and veins
- defects in the partitions between the atria or the ventricles.

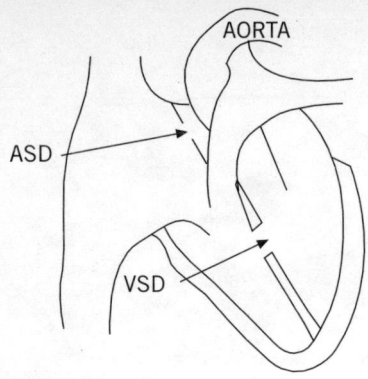

The most common of these defects are:

- *Atrial septal defect (ASD)* An opening between the two atria (the top cardiac chambers) caused by a hole in the atrial septum.
- *Ventricular septal defect (VSD)* An opening between the two ventricles (the lower cardiac chambers) caused by a hole in the ventricular septum.
- *Pulmonary stenosis (PS)* A narrowing of the valve leading to the lungs.
- *Patent ductus arteriosus (PDA)* A connection between the aorta and the pulmonary artery, which usually closes at birth, remains open.
- *Coarctation of the aorta* A narrowing of the aorta, the main blood vessel leading from the heart.

The treatment for congenital heart disorders is usually surgery.

Electrical problems (rhythm disorders)

Just as a mechanical pump requires a power supply, so our hearts have a system of electrical impulses that control the heart muscle's ability to contract and expand. The source of this electrical 'supply' is found in the right atrium and is called the *sinus node* – our body's natural pacemaker.

Arrhythmia

Quite simply this is a long word which means a heartbeat that is irregular or abnormally fast or slow. It is not uncommon for many of us to experience an irregular heartbeat, though if it remains

THE HEART AND THE THINGS THAT CAN GO WRONG

persistent it could be an indicator of heart disease and should be mentioned to your doctor.

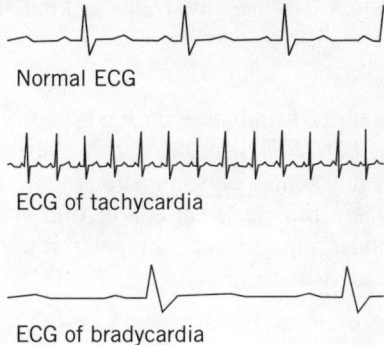

There are three main categories of arrhythmia:
- tachycardia: a rapid heartbeat
- bradycardia: a slow heartbeat
- fibrillation: an irregular heartbeat.

The symptoms of arrhythmia are palpitations, a racing or pounding heart, dizziness, sudden fainting spells.

Arrhythmias can be either in the atria or the ventricles, although ventricular arrhythmias tend to be more serious.

> **Ectopic beats**
>
> Our hearts, ever conscious of our welfare, have spare back-up pacemakers in the chambers of the heart which can be triggered off to give what are called 'ectopic beats'.

Atrial arrhythmias
- Atrial ectopic beats – extra heartbeats from the atrium – can feel like a dropped beat.
- Atrial tachycardias – the atria start to race, usually about 140–160 beats per minute. This is called supraventricular tachycardia (SVT). This can often be stopped by lying down with your feet raised above the height of your head.
- Atrial fibrillation – the atria are beating fast and irregularly.

Ventricular arrhythmias
- Ventricular ectopic beats – there are additional beats from the ventricles.

- Ventricular tachycardia – the ventricles beat very fast. This can be a very dangerous rhythm.
- Ventricular fibrillation – the ventricles are quivering instead of beating. This causes cardiac arrest and is fatal if not stopped – usually with a defibrillator.

Slow heartbeats
- Bradycardia – a super-fit athlete can have a very slow heartbeat (40 per minute), but slow heartbeats can also occur with heart disease, or from the action of some drugs.
- Heart block – where the electrical conduction system is blocked, and the sinus node impulses cannot get through. Sometimes a pacemaker is needed to fix this.

Pacemakers

If your heartbeat slows right down to less than 30–35 beats per minute or you have episodes when your natural pacemaker, the sinus node, stops, you will more than likely be fitted with an artificial pacemaker.

The pacemaker is small, discus shaped and about the size of a squashed golf ball. It is very easily inserted using local anaesthetic, placed under the skin and below the collarbone. Attached to it is a fine wire that is fed into a vein and passed into the inside of the heart, where it sits and waits for the heartbeats to slow. If they do, it sends a signal to the heart, telling it to go back to normal.

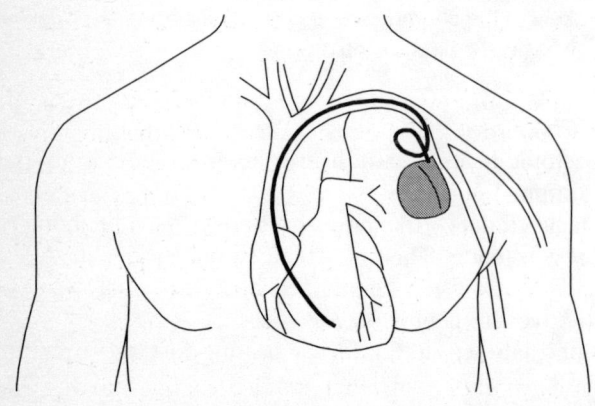

THE HEART AND THE THINGS THAT CAN GO WRONG

For most people the fitting of a pacemaker is a very minor procedure with only minimal discomfort. Once it is in place you'll forget about it, not knowing whether it's working or just waiting to do its job. However, just knowing it's there is immensely reassuring.

> **Palpitations**
>
> At some time or another most of us will experience palpitations, that rather scary awareness of our heartbeat. It could be that we have an electrical problem, but more than likely they are a result of overindulgence in coffee or alcohol, smoking or plain old-fashioned anxiety. If you experience palpitations more than infrequently it would pay you to see your doctor who may ask you to have Holter monitoring (see Holter monitoring, p. 33).

Valve problems

Our hard-working little pump has within it four valves which regulate the blood flow through our heart – these are called the mitral, aortic, tricuspid and pulmonary valves.

As blood flows through each of the heart's four chambers it is the valves opening and closing that give us the familiar sound of our heartbeat.

The valves usually work perfectly, letting blood pass from one heart chamber to the next. Occasionally they can malfunction, become narrow or leak and allow the blood to flow in the wrong direction. This can result in more strain on the heart and in some instances eventually cause heart failure.

- *Mitral valve prolapse* This is a common valve complaint that is caused when a valve has an excess of tissue that prevents it from closing fully. In most cases this condition can be corrected by surgery, although it is quite common for many people to lead normal, active lives without the need for either surgery or medication.
- *Narrowing (stenosis) of the aortic or mitral valve* Because the heart has to work extra hard, narrowing of these valves can sometimes cause heart failure and/or angina.
- *Valve regurgitation* In other words, leaking valves. These can also increase the heart's workload and cause heart failure.

Infective endocarditis

Throughout our lives our bodies are host to bacteria and normally our immune system will prevent any build-up causing damage. However, when a valve is damaged it tends to attract a build-up of bacteria, which can cause an infection that in turn will further damage the affected valve.

Treatment of infective endocarditis is usually aggressive – a course of intravenous antibiotics – or in some cases surgery may be necessary.

Stroke

The term 'stroke' is used to describe a number of events that occur when blood supply to the brain is obstructed. When an artery supplying blood to any section of the brain becomes blocked, the area that is supplied will die and the body functions for which that part of the brain is responsible will cease.

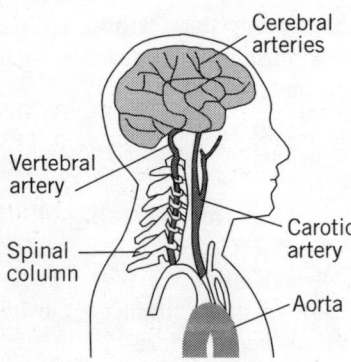

There are three basic forms of stroke:
- *Cerebral thrombosis*, when blood flow to the brain is blocked by a clot which develops in one of the cerebral arteries.
- *Cerebral embolism*, when a piece of plaque that is attached to the lining of a blood vessel, or a clot within the heart, breaks free and lodges in a cerebral artery.
- *Cerebral haemorrhage*, which occurs when a cerebral artery bursts and bleeds into the brain.

TIAs (transient ischaemic attacks)

These are brief, stroke-like symptoms that last for just a few seconds or minutes. As angina is a warning sign that all is not well with the heart, so these 'mini-strokes' – TIAs – should be regarded as a serious warning that a stroke may occur in the future.

Do not ignore these warning signs – see your doctor urgently. (See Appendix B – Suggested reading, p. 103.)

Symptoms of a stroke

Because of the damage done to the brain, any sign of a stroke should be treated as a serious medical emergency. Symptoms – which are likely to appear suddenly – include the following:

- a feeling of numbness in the face, arm and leg on one side of the body
- loss or deterioration of speech, sight or feeling
- memory loss and confusion
- dizziness and loss of balance
- sudden and severe headache.

Diabetes

If you have diabetes the chances of your developing some form of heart disease are about double that of the general population. It is therefore imperative that anyone with diabetes, whatever their age, pay particular attention to the welfare of their heart.

What is diabetes?

Diabetes is a disease where too much sugar accumulates in the bloodstream, rather than being used by cells throughout the body. It's not that you get diabetes from eating too much sugar, it's more that your body doesn't produce enough insulin – the hormone that allows the sugar (glucose) to enter the cells and produce energy.

There are two types of diabetes: either your body doesn't make sufficient insulin or it can't respond properly to the insulin that it does make.

Type 1   The body makes little or no insulin and insulin injections are essential to maintain life.

Type 2   The body is making insulin but it is failing to use it properly. This is the more common type of diabetes and can often be controlled by regular exercise and a healthy eating programme, although sometimes medication is needed.

Recent evidence suggests that, all things being equal, women with diabetes are more at risk of developing heart disease than men. (See Appendix B – Suggested reading, p. 103.)

> **Symptoms of Diabetes**
>
> *Type 1*   The initial symptoms usually appear quite suddenly.
>
> - increased thirst
> - more frequent urination
> - tiredness
> - weight loss – despite increased eating.
>
> *Type 2*   Symptoms develop more slowly and may include any of the above except weight loss in addition to the following.
>
> - frequent or slow-to-heal infections, particularly of the skin, gum or bladder
> - blurred vision
> - tingling or numbness of the hands or feet.
>
> These three symptoms can also occur later in type 1 diabetes.

Heart attack (myocardial infarction – MI)

Any sudden blockage of blood flowing through the coronary artery that causes damage to the heart muscle or tissue is called a heart attack. The technical name you will often hear your doctor use is *myocardial infarction* or *MI*, which comes from the two words *myocardium* – the heart muscle and *infarction* – the death of tissue. Because it is the coronary arteries that are involved, a heart attack is sometimes called simply 'a coronary'.

The heart muscle, while starved of blood, is often damaged and left with scarred muscle tissue. Such scarring can cause a number of problems:
- *Electrical*   Many rhythm disturbances, from benign additional beats to serious ventricular tachycardia and fibrillation which causes cardiac arrest (see p. 21).
- *Pumping*   If too much of the heart muscle is damaged, the heart cannot work properly and heart failure can develop.

THE HEART AND THE THINGS THAT CAN GO WRONG

What to do if you think you're having a heart attack

In reality you're not going to have time to find this book and refer to this section so we would advise that you study it and try to remember as much as possible.

- Stay as calm as you can.
- Call 999, ask for the ambulance service, and tell them you have chest pain. If you're not up to it get someone else to make this call.
- Try to be clear in telling the operator what is wrong and where you are.
- Sit comfortably, loosen your clothing, try to relax and breathe deeply and slowly.
- If you have a glyceryl trinitrate spray or tablet, use it and repeat every 5 minutes.
- If possible chew and swallow an aspirin.

DO NOT!

- Be embarrassed in case it's only heartburn.
- Wait to see if the pain goes away.
- Be concerned about putting anyone out.
- Think you're too young to have a heart attack.
- Try to drive yourself to the hospital.

Remember . . .

The sooner you get assistance the less chance there is of any damage being done. The ambulance staff are proud of what they do and would rather deal with a false alarm than a dead or dying body.

Warning signs of a heart attack

The classic signs that you are having, or are about to have, a heart attack are not easy to ignore. Whether the symptoms come on suddenly or are a growing, nagging discomfort, do not hesitate – *call an ambulance immediately.*

The symptoms are:

- a strong persistent pressure across the chest, as if an elephant were sitting on it
- pain radiating to your shoulders, back, neck, lower jaw, and down your arm

- a burning sensation in the upper abdomen
- shortness of breath, nausea, sweating
- anxiety and fatigue.

What to do if someone else is having a heart attack

If you are present when someone else is having a heart attack the best thing you can do is help them follow the above procedures. If the person cannot be roused and you know how to administer CPR (cardiopulmonary resuscitation) do so as soon as possible. If you don't know CPR you may find a passer-by who can help.

A heart attack, while understandably frightening, should be taken as a warning, and you should look at changing your lifestyle. (See Beating the odds, p. 45.)

After the heart attack

All going to plan, you will find yourself in the safe hands of the hospital. First you'll be taken to Accident and Emergency (A&E) where they will immediately confirm your condition and take steps to stabilize you and make you comfortable.

- While the staff ask questions about your symptoms and past medical history they will attach electrocardiogram (ECG) electrodes to monitor your heart rhythm. (See ECG, p. 35.)
- An intravenous line will be inserted into your arm so that, should the need arise, you can immediately be given the appropriate medication.
- If necessary you will be given a clot-busting drug to clear any blockage that is causing the heart attack.
- Blood samples will be taken and sent to the laboratory for analysis.
- You will be given various medications to ease any pain, decrease the clotting, improve the heart rate and lower your blood pressure.
- By monitoring your heart rhythm, any dangerous change can be detected and rapidly reversed. Cardiac arrest due to ventricular fibrillation is quite common early in a heart attack, and can be easily treated with defibrillation – but only if a defibrillator is available. This is why you need to get to an ambulance or hospital as quickly as possible.

THE HEART AND THE THINGS THAT CAN GO WRONG

Once you are stable you will probably be taken to a specialized unit in the hospital called the *coronary care unit* (CCU) where a team of doctors and nurses will monitor your condition and start you on the road to recovery.

Depending on the outcome of the tests, further procedures such as an angiogram or ultrasound may be ordered (see pp. 31–37). It's also possible that you may be asked to undergo an exercise stress test (see Stress test, p. 34).

The average stay in the CCU is normally two or three days – shorter if it wasn't a heart attack, but longer if there are complications. Frequently you then go to a step-down ward and when the doctors think it's safe for you to go home, you will be discharged into the care of your doctor and a further appointment made with the hospital for some time in the near future.

When you get home think about what's happened: you've had a warning, and you must now begin the journey not only to recovery but also to a healthier and more fulfilling life. (See Beating the odds, p. 45.)

Cardiac arrest (sudden cardiac death)

This is not another name for a heart attack but is a condition caused by a fault in the heart's electrical system which causes the heart muscles to stop (arrest). When the heart stops beating the blood flow through the body stops and no oxygen can reach the brain. This results in unconsciousness and unless resuscitation is started immediately, the result is nearly always fatal.

There are no specific warning symptoms indicating cardiac arrest, but it occurs most commonly early after a heart attack, although it can occur without any warning at all. Indeed, for many people, cardiac arrest is the first warning that they have heart disease, and sadly in most cases the last. This is why early detection of heart disease is so important.

THE HEART AND THE THINGS THAN CAN GO WRONG

> **Common causes of cardiac arrest**
>
> - Heart attack – most cardiac arrests are caused by heart attacks but they can also occur through . . .
> - drowning
> - drug overdose
> - electric shock
> - suffocation
> - trauma.

CPR (cardiopulmonary resuscitation)

When our hearts stop pumping, the brain and body will die unless someone steps in to help. CPR (cardiopulmonary resuscitation or heart–lung resuscitation) is a skill all adults and young people should learn. It is easy and can save a life. This life could be that of your partner, parent or another loved one – or even a stranger. Heart massage and mouth-to-mouth respiration can keep a victim alive until the ambulance arrives with a defibrillator.

If someone close to you has a heart condition you may like to learn how to apply CPR. The British Heart Foundation funds the Heartstart UK initiative, and St John Ambulance runs a range of courses including CPR (see Appendix C – Useful addresses, p. 105).

Defibrillation is the only way to get the heart back into a useful rhythm. The earlier it is done the more likely it is to be successful. (See p. 20.)

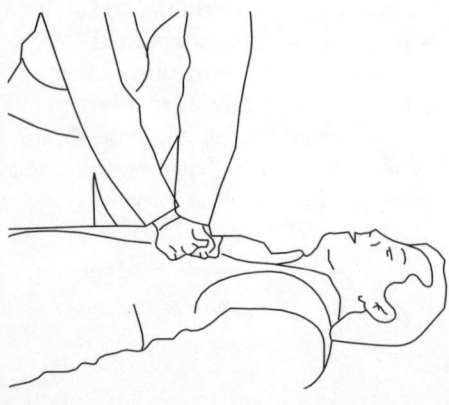

THE HEART AND THE THINGS THAT CAN GO WRONG

Defibrillation

This is a procedure we've seen dozens of times on television and in the movies, when our screen doctor uses a sophisticated piece of equipment to 'jump start' a heart that has stopped beating. And so it is in real life: an electric current is delivered to the heart in order to shock it into its normal rhythm.

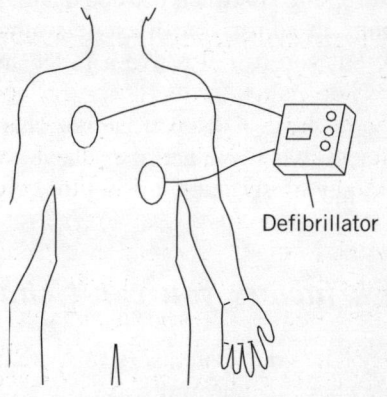

Defibrillator

Don't be a tough guy *Studies have shown that self-disclosure – talking about your feelings – certainly helps you confront and manage what it is that is the cause of your concern.*

2
So who's at risk?

> Man is not the creature of circumstances.
> Circumstances are the creatures of men.
> Benjamin Disraeli, *Vivian Grey* (1826–27)

Knowing and understanding the risk factors involved in heart disease could make the difference between life and death. Being aware gives you the opportunity to adjust your lifestyle so that not only are the risks minimized, but you can also live a fuller and more enjoyable life.

Though there are some risks you cannot change, just knowing what they are, and what impact they have on your life, can encourage you to pay closer attention to those risk factors you can change.

Risk factors you can't change

- *Family history* If your parents, grandparents or other close family members have had heart disease you have a greater chance of being at risk.
- *Age* As we get older our chances of being diagnosed with heart disease become greater. Over 75 per cent of people who die from coronary artery disease are aged 65 or older.
- *Gender* Men are more likely to suffer a heart attack than women, particularly in early life. (See Men's hearts – women's hearts, p. 4.) After menopause, women start to catch up.
- *Race* The incidence of heart disease among different ethnic groupings varies enormously. In New Zealand Maori and Pacific Islanders have a much higher rate of heart disease than Caucasians, who are themselves more at risk than the Asian or Oriental community. But countries with previously low levels of heart disease (Japan, India and eastern Europe) are experiencing an increase in heart disease as they embrace a Western lifestyle and diet.
- *Diabetes* For people with diabetes there is an increased chance of developing coronary artery disease. Anyone with diabetes is advised to pay particular attention to minimizing those risk factors that they have control over. (See Diabetes, p. 17.)

SO WHO'S AT RISK?
Risk factors you can change

If any of the unavoidable risks apply to you, then you should pay particular attention to those risks you can control.

Diet

One of the key elements in reducing the risk of heart disease is eating a balanced diet of the food that is good for your heart. Over the last few decades the incidence of heart disease has risen faster than at any time in the past. Why? Because the modern Western diet encourages the development of heart disease.

Get your diet right and you'll go a long way towards preventing heart disease. If you have been diagnosed as having heart disease then the correct diet, in conjunction with reducing other risk factors, can hold the disease in check and may even reverse the damage already done.

There is a great truth in the saying that we are what we eat. And when you think about it, doesn't it make sense? Unfortunately, we in the West have become seduced into eating a diet that is heavy with animal fats and these, as we now know, are what contribute to the unacceptably high incidence of heart disease in our society.

But it needn't be so; there are any number of alternative foods and recipes that are not only healthier but will also make us feel better. (See We are what we eat, p. 54.)

Blood cholesterol

Cholesterol is an essential building block in many of our body's cells and hormones. We produce it in our liver, as well as absorb it into our system from the animal foods we eat. However, excessive amounts of cholesterol in the blood contribute to the build-up of plaque in our arteries, which in turn can lead to coronary artery disease (CAD). (See Coronary artery disease, p. 5.)

Good and bad cholesterol

Because cholesterol cannot dissolve in water or blood, it is carried through our circulatory system in tiny shells called lipoproteins.

Shells carrying cholesterol to our tissues are called low-density lipoprotein (LDL); those returning cholesterol back to the liver for cleaning are called high-density lipoprotein (HDL).

SO WHO'S AT RISK?

Bad cholesterol (LDL) contributes to the build-up of the plaque that narrows the arteries. Good cholesterol (HDL) removes any excess of bad cholesterol and thus lowers the risk of coronary artery disease.

It is important that we get the balance right between good and bad cholesterol.

Your cholesterol readings

If you are thought to be at risk of heart disease one of the first tests your doctor will ask for is a full lipid profile blood test from a medical laboratory. Such a test will clearly show your levels of both good and bad cholesterol, as well as the level of your blood triglycerides. Triglycerides are the carriers of fat around the body and high levels increase the risk of coronary artery disease.

Homocysteine

Recent studies have indicated that high levels of homocysteine (an amino acid) in the blood may increase the risk of developing blocked arteries. It is thought that this may be caused by a low level of vitamins B6, B12 and folic acid in the diet. In some countries (including Australia and the USA) folic acid is being added to wheat and flour to keep levels of homocysteine down. To be on the safe side you should include these vitamins as part of your diet. (See We are what we eat, p. 54.)

What the readings mean

Cholesterol levels are shown as millimoles per litre (mmol/l).
  Acceptable readings are:

- *Total cholesterol* 3.0–5.0 mmol/l
- *LDL* Bad cholesterol – should be as low as possible, preferably in the 2–3 mmol/l range
- *HDL* Good cholesterol – needs to be as high as possible, preferably over 1 mmol/l
- *Triglycerides* Less than 2.0 mmol/l
- *Other tests* Lipoprotein (a) (abbreviated as Lp(a)), and Apolipoprotein B are also undesirable, and need to be as low as possible

---

Lower your cholesterol levels

We now know that the levels of cholesterol in our blood greatly contribute to the risk of our having heart disease. So we have to get our levels of both good and bad cholesterol just right. Here's how we can do it:

- Eat the right foods (see We are what we eat, p. 54).
- Exercise – the 30 minutes that will help lower your blood pressure will at the same time help increase your good cholesterol level (see Keeping the body moving, p. 70).
- Medication – your doctor will advise you on this (see Appendix A – The drugs we take, p. 95).
- Stop smoking (see p. 28).

High blood pressure

In most cases there is no known cause of high blood pressure, but for many of us the stresses of modern twenty-first century living make it worse (see Hypertension, p. 9).

Because high blood pressure makes the heart work harder and can contribute to heart disease it is advisable to keep it under control.

Reduce your blood pressure

High blood pressure is a 'silent killer'. Here's what you should look out for.

- *Smoking* Any form of tobacco smoke will increase your blood pressure. The good news is that soon after you stop smoking you'll begin to feel the benefits.
- *Keep an eye on your weight* You'd be surprised how even a few kilos lost from the right places can make a difference.
- *Salt* Cut it back slowly and you'll soon train your palate to get used to a healthier diet (see We are what we eat, p. 54).
- *Alcohol* A glass or two of wine a day will most probably do you more good than harm. But beware – more than two glasses will raise your blood pressure and could do you harm (see We are what we eat, p. 54).
- *Lack of exercise* All you need is at least 30 minutes five or six days a week and you'll be doing wonders for yourself (see Keeping the body moving, p. 70).
- *Stress* If you are overanxious about things you'll more than likely get stressed and that will put your blood pressure up. Try to learn how to manage the anxiety and stress in your life. Look at the medical word for high blood pressure – hypertension. 'Hyper' means too much and 'tension' speaks for itself (see Coping with stress, p. 75).

Note If lifestyle changes do not lower your blood pressure enough, then your doctor may decide to start you on blood pressure-lowering drugs. (See Appendix A – The drugs we take, p. 95.)

The 'couch potato' syndrome

The human body, like all sophisticated machinery, needs to be kept active – especially the heart, which depends on exercise to keep it healthy and strong. The benefits of a regular exercise regime are that it:

- helps lower blood pressure
- increases the body's production of good cholesterol (HDL)
- improves the heart's ability to use oxygen more efficiently
- encourages weight loss
- makes you feel much healthier – because you are!

Get off your backside!

We have not developed over the last few million years by lazing around doing little or no physical exercise. Our bodies need exercise – not a lot, but some! How much you need and the best way to go about getting it is covered in our section on exercise. (See Keeping the body moving, p. 70.)

Stress

Stress, like heart disease, is a condition of our times. It raises the level of adrenalin in the blood which in turn has many effects on our heart: blood pressure rises, our heart rate increases, blood vessels can narrow, cholesterol levels may increase and our blood becomes stickier and can clot more easily.

Though we may not do away with all the stress in our lives – and after all, we do need some, it's what motivates and drives us – there is much we can do to contain and manage it. (See Coping with stress, p. 75.)

Smoking

If you are a smoker you are up to four times more likely to develop coronary artery disease than non-smokers and 70 per cent more at risk of it being fatal. We know that smoking damages the lungs, but why is it bad for the heart?

SO WHO'S AT RISK?

- It increases heart rate and blood pressure, making the heart work harder to supply oxygen to the rest of your body.
- Tobacco smoke produces carbon monoxide, which reduces the blood's oxygen-carrying ability.
- It damages your artery linings, making them more susceptible to narrowing and hardening.
- It increases bad cholesterol and decreases the good.
- It causes emphysema and a number of rather nasty cancers.
- Women who smoke tend to have lower than normal oestrogen – the hormone that protects against heart disease.

Smoking and women
For reasons that we don't quite understand, women who have a history of even mild smoking are more at risk than male smokers.

Passive smoking
This means taking into your body other people's smoke. It is also a powerful risk factor, particularly for young children who are brought up by parents who smoke. If other people start smoking in front of you, politely but very firmly ask them not to – your health is too important.

> **Just a thought . . .** *If you smoke 20 cigarettes a day, and let's say you started when you were 20 and you're now 40, do you realize that you've spent over £25,000 on killing yourself? Think what you'd have now if you had saved and invested that money. Shame.*

Damage done by smoking may never be reversed.
For further information on how you can cut down your risk of developing heart disease please refer to the 'Let's get healthy' plan on p. 46.

> **Reward yourself.** *A silly little thing really but you'll be surprised at how well it works. All you have to do is work out a number of ways you'll treat yourself every time you eat or do something you're really not that mad about. Better still, get your family to decide what is best for you to be rewarded for – and make the reward for all the family, maybe a night out or a long-wanted CD.*

SO WHO'S AT RISK?

Some suggestions for stopping smoking

- Prepare yourself for quitting: set a special day, perhaps a birthday or an anniversary.
- Read as much information on stopping smoking as you can.
- Involve a friend – perhaps there's someone who'll quit with you.
- Be realistic – you will have withdrawal symptoms, but they do go away.
- Work out when you tend to smoke and learn what triggers you to light up.
- Try to avoid those situations when you do light up.
- See smoking as a negative thing – it smells, it's disgusting and it's costing you an awful lot of money.
- What could you buy with what you save from not smoking?
- If you feel restless – and you will – go for a walk; it'll do you good as well.
- Some people find taking up a hobby that keeps their hands busy can be very helpful.
- Magnesium can help reduce that nagging, craving feeling.
- If you have a relapse, think of it as a learning experience.

3
What the doctors can do

> A disease known is half cured.
> Thomas Fuller MD, *Gnomologia* (1732)

If your GP suspects that all is not well with your heart he/she may refer you to a cardiologist (a doctor who specializes in diseases of the heart). The cardiologist will ask you questions, give you a physical examination and most likely ask for a series of tests to be done. These tests are to give your doctor the information needed to tell exactly what is wrong with you.

The tests you'll have

Questions and the physical examination

Diagnostic examinations begin with you being asked:

- your symptoms – why are you there?
- your past medical history
- any medication you are taking, and any allergies
- your family's medical history.

After these questions the next step is a physical examination. Your doctor will be looking for the following:

- The veins in your neck. These give similar information to a dipstick in your car: they tell if you have too much or too little fluid in the circulation, and also show the pressures in the heart.
- Does the skin feel warm or cold, and what is its colour?
- Are the ankles swollen, suggesting heart failure? Feeling the size of the liver, at the top right of your abdomen, can also suggest this.
- Is your pulse even or erratic, and how fast is it going?
- Are your lungs clear or do they contain excess fluid?
- What is your blood pressure?

The findings of the physical examination will determine the nature of any further tests you may be asked to have.

Describing your symptoms

The better your doctor understands how you are feeling, the better he/she will be able to help you. We all tend to fumble around a bit at the doctor's, so before you go to the surgery consider these points and write them down as a reminder:

- What is it that you feel?
- Where does it bother you?
- How bad is it?
- What brings it on?
- How does it come on – gradually or suddenly?
- Does anything reduce or eliminate it?
- How long has it been happening?
- How long does it last?

Note Also think of any little things that aren't quite right, not just the obvious ones. The more the doctor knows, the more accurate the diagnosis will be.

The stethoscope – cardiac auscultation

One of the oldest means of diagnosis, the stethoscope, lets your doctor hear how your heart sounds. In some conditions there are additional noises and murmurs, which can indicate that something is not right. The stethoscope can also assess the state of the lungs and see if they contain too much fluid.

Blood tests

Blood tests can help your doctors to diagnose certain cardiac conditions and thus decide on the best treatment. Blood tests are used to:

- detect signs of a heart attack and damage to the heart muscle by measuring the cardiac enzymes and troponins
- measure your cholesterol levels
- measure the minerals that can affect heart function – sodium,

potassium, calcium and magnesium; check that your kidneys and liver are working satisfactorily
- uncover any tendency there may be for diabetes.

X-rays

An X-ray of your chest can indicate an enlarged heart or a build-up of fluid in the lungs, both signs of possible heart failure.

ECG (electrocardiogram)

Having an ECG is painless. It monitors your heart rhythm while you're resting and records the electrical pattern as the heart beats. To the trained eye it will show:

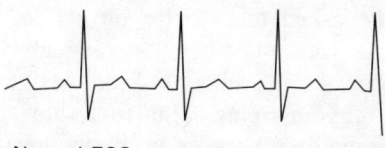

Normal ECG

- abnormalities in your heart's electrical impulses and abnormal rhythms
- evidence of thickening of the heart wall
- signs of a previous heart attack.

If there are indications that the heart rhythm may be abnormal, you may be asked to wear a Holter monitor (see below) which will give a clearer picture of any underlying problem.

Holter monitoring

A small, portable ECG monitor worn for 24 hours that gives a continuous reading of the heartbeat. When the wearer experiences any abnormality a button can be pressed to mark the sensation so that it can later be matched to the printed reading.

Stress test (also referred to as an exercise test)

A stress test is just what it says – a test to see how your heart responds when you exert physical stress on it. You will be connected to an ECG (see above) and a reading will be taken and noted while you are at rest. The team conducting the test will then place you on either a treadmill or an exercise bicycle and gradually increase the level of exercise. The aim is usually for you to exercise for as long as you can or to get the heart rate to a predicted level. You will be closely monitored and the test stopped if there are any abnormal readings. You can also stop the test at any time you feel undue discomfort.

The printed readings will give a fair indication of the diagnosis and whether further tests are necessary.

Thallium stress test (also called a perfusion scan)

This is a test that assesses heart function and blood flow through the coronary arteries to your heart muscle.

You will first be asked to exercise on a treadmill or exercise bicycle for as long as you can. When you've reached your maximum and can go no further, a small amount of radioactive thallium will be injected into one of your veins. This is a safe and tiny dose of irradiation, and the thallium is taken up by the heart as blood flows to it. Areas which have a poor blood flow will show less radioactivity, which is seen by a special nuclear camera. If you've previously experienced a heart attack this test will also show the areas of damage.

Ultrasound (echocardiography)

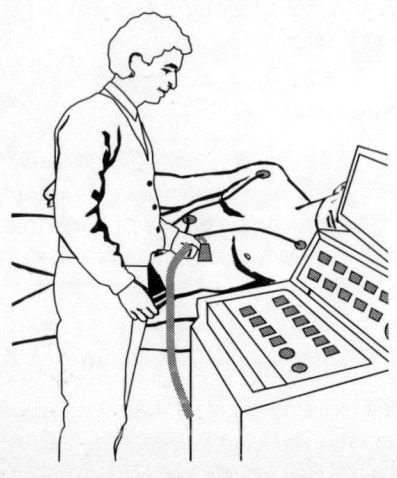

WHAT THE DOCTORS CAN DO

An echocardiogram uses high-frequency sound waves to create a picture of the working heart (you have most probably seen it or heard about it being used more commonly to show the foetus during pregnancy).

Ultrasound has a wide range of diagnostic uses:

- to evaluate how well the heart is working
- to see how the blood flows through the heart
- to identify any damage to the heart muscle or the heart itself
- to determine the presence of valve disease
- to follow the progress of valve disease
- to determine the presence of congenital heart disease (see p. 11).

CT or CAT scan (computerized tomography)

This test uses computer processing together with X-ray imaging. New ultrafast CT scanners are now being used to determine the levels of calcium in the coronary arteries which may allow early diagnosis of coronary artery disease.

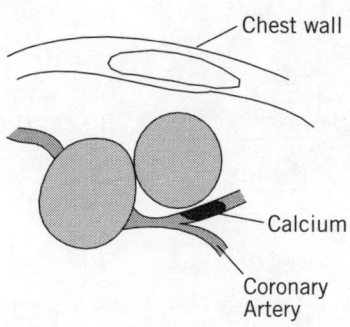

Angiography (catheterization)

This is the name given to a procedure where a small, hollow, flexible tube (a catheter) is inserted into an artery or vein in the thigh or arm and is then threaded through into the arteries or chambers of the heart. Scary though it may sound, the movement of the catheter

WHAT THE DOCTORS CAN DO

usually causes no sensations, and local anaesthetic of the skin where the catheter is inserted is all that is needed. Catheterization is used:

- To show the arteries, indicate where they go, and see if there is any narrowing or blockage. When examining the heart arteries this is called *coronary angiography*.
- To measure the pressures and blood flow within the heart; sometimes the amount of oxygen is tested in the chambers to detect congenital heart defects.
- To assess valve performance – both narrowing or leaking.

Although you will be given a mild sedative to help you relax, you will remain awake for the procedure. The doctor will use X-ray equipment to guide the catheter into the heart or coronary arteries. Once the catheter is in place, a special dye is introduced which is visible on an X-ray and will clearly show if there is narrowing or blockage of the arteries. An *angiogram* is the name given to the X-ray photo that records the condition of your arteries.

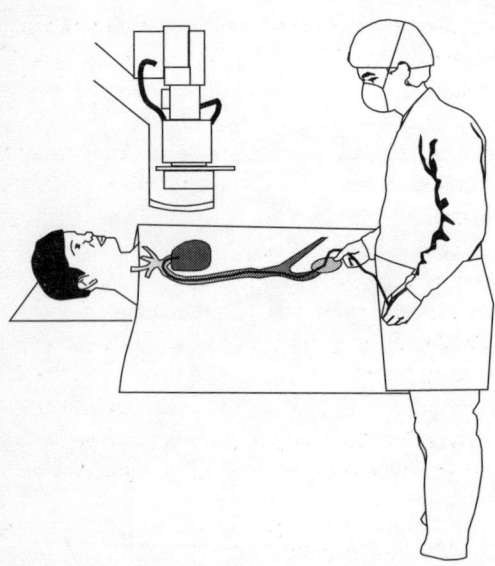

Note The dye that is used sometimes contains iodine, so you will be asked to confirm that you are not allergic to iodine.

WHAT THE DOCTORS CAN DO

After the tests

After all the tests have been completed and the results are in, your GP and cardiologist will know exactly what's wrong with you and can set in motion the treatment that will put you on the road to recovery.

Medication

Unless there has been a complete false alarm the chances are that you'll be prescribed a course of medication. Perhaps that's as far as it will go for the moment, other than a watchful eye being kept on you.

Safe use of medication

- Make sure you understand the medication that you're on and why it's been prescribed. If your doctor doesn't explain – ASK!
- Tell your doctor if you are on any other, non-heart medication, or if you are taking supplements.
- Find out at what time of the day your medication should be taken and whether this should be before, after or with food.
- If you forget to take your medication, DO NOT double up. Consult your doctor or pharmacist.
- Some medication can cause side-effects – learn what these are; if you experience them and they persist, tell your doctor. There is almost always an alternative.
- Tell your doctor of any unusual effects you experience.
- Check if your medication prohibits drinking alcohol.
- Keep your medication in its original containers.
- Keep a list of your medicines and take it with you whenever you see your doctor.
- Do not offer your medicines to others or take theirs.
- If you visit your dentist tell him/her what medication you are on.
- Make sure you take a supply of your medicines when going on holiday.

Keep medicines away from children.

Aspirin

With our modern reliance on technology it is hard to believe that one of the great fighters against heart disease is a natural product that comes from the bark of the willow tree and has been around for over 100 years – acetylsalicylic acid, or aspirin.

It doesn't, as is commonly believed, 'thin' the blood, but rather it makes the platelets that build up as plaque in the arteries less sticky and less prone to build up and cause clots. Most people with coronary artery disease should be taking aspirin daily.

A low dose of aspirin (between 75 and 100 mg daily) is all that is needed. Many aspirin preparations have a special enteric coating that prevents the aspirin from being released in your stomach, where it could cause the gastric upsets you may have experienced with uncoated aspirin. The aspirin is released lower down in the intestine, from where it is absorbed gradually into the bloodstream.

Note Talk to your doctor about whether you should be taking aspirin and about dosage – too high a dose can be dangerous.

Angioplasty and stents

For most people diagnosed with heart disease, the blockages can be treated with medication and changes in lifestyle. However, if your cardiologist feels that your heart disease is likely to put you at risk or if your symptoms cannot easily be controlled with medication, there are two further options – angioplasty and surgery.

Angioplasty (coronary or balloon angioplasty)

If your arteries show significant blocking, your consultant may decide that the best course of action is to open up the blockage using angioplasty.

This is a procedure similar to catheterization (see p. 35). A long, narrow tube with a small high-pressure balloon at its end is inserted through a blood vessel in the thigh up to and beyond the point of the blockage. When in place the balloon is inflated for 15–60 seconds, squeezing the plaque against the artery wall, opening up the artery and allowing a better flow of blood (see below).

WHAT THE DOCTORS CAN DO

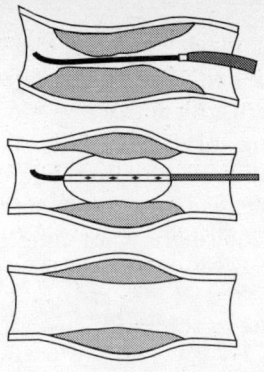

Stents

In many cases your doctor may also wish to insert a stent. After the artery has been opened by the balloon, a small, expanding, wire-mesh tube (stent) is inserted in the blockage, then expanded, and left holding the artery open.

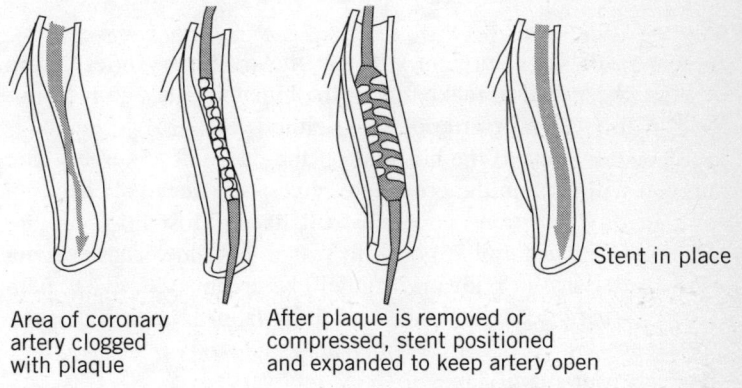

Area of coronary artery clogged with plaque

After plaque is removed or compressed, stent positioned and expanded to keep artery open

Stent in place

Surgery

If your angiogram (see above) shows a number of blockages or if the main coronary artery is diseased, your cardiologist may recommend that you have a surgical procedure called coronary artery bypass graft surgery (CABG) – commonly known as open heart surgery or just simply as a bypass.

WHAT THE DOCTORS CAN DO
Coronary artery bypass graft surgery (CABG)

This is a surgical procedure where arterial blockages are bypassed by grafts – either arteries or veins taken from other areas in your body. It is performed by a heart surgeon. During the operation you will be placed on a heart–lung machine which takes over the blood circulation so the heart can be stopped while the bypass vessels are attached. New techniques can now allow surgeons to operate on a beating heart without requiring a heart–lung bypass.

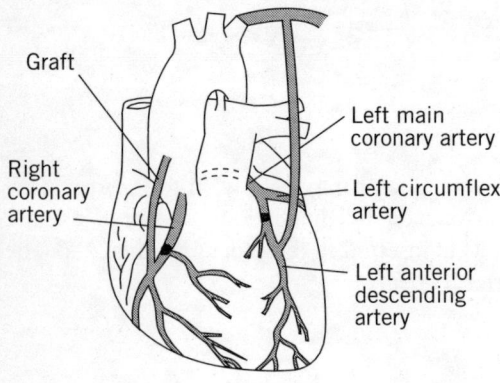

In most cases your surgeon will use the mammary artery from inside your chest wall to make one of the bypasses, though it is also possible to use veins or arteries from either your arm or leg.

You'll be admitted to the hospital on the day before surgery and the surgeon will explain the procedure, give you your final check-up and answer any questions you may still have. Most hospitals are quite happy for your family to be with you at this time. That evening a nurse will shave your body and you will be given a sedative to help you sleep. Generally surgery takes anything from four to six hours, during which time you will be fully anaesthetized.

There are four main stages to your recovery:

1 The intensive care unit (ICU)
This is where you'll be for the first 24–48 hours after your surgery. You'll be very woozy and the chances are you won't remember much about it at all. Your family will be able to visit, although you should warn them that they may find it disturbing because of the many tubes and wires that will still be attached to you. This is quite normal and is nothing to worry about.

WHAT THE DOCTORS CAN DO

2 The post-surgery ward

Once the doctors are happy that all is stable you'll be moved into the post-surgery ward where you'll stay for the next four to six days. Because of the trauma of the surgery you are likely to be somewhat depressed and most probably a little irritable. *This is a very normal reaction which will soon pass.*

The nurses and physiotherapists will get you on your feet and moving about pretty quickly to speed up your recovery. Your appetite, which has most probably left you, will return and very soon you'll be back to eating good food.

3 Going home

For the first few weeks after you get home it's quite natural for you to feel disoriented and tired. The hospital will have given you information on your recovery programme and you should start getting mobile as soon as possible. Begin with five minutes' slow walking five times a day and slowly build on that. If you find you get tired or short of breath – stop, take a rest and start again a little later.

Many people after a short time at home begin to get feelings of frustration, anger, fear and depression – it's very normal and will pass, so don't try to be a hero – talk about it with your family and tell your doctor.

4 The rest of your life

You've had your operation, you're up and about and life is getting back to normal. You have no more angina, the doctors have taken you off much of your medication and you're feeling pretty happy with life, the universe and everything. Well, that's fine and good luck to you – but don't get too carried away. You may feel better than you have in a long time, but the underlying cause of what was wrong is still there – you had heart disease *and you still have heart disease*. The doctors, nurses and surgeons have fixed the effect – but they can't fix the cause. It's now up to you.

How to hold your condition in check – and maybe even reverse it – is fully covered in Living with heart disease, p. 54.

WHAT THE DOCTORS CAN DO

> **Common feelings after bypass surgery**
>
> Following their surgery most patients notice a number of strange changes:
>
> - They become very emotional – tears appear very easily.
> - They feel the cold more than they used to.
> - They notice their heart beating more than before.
> - They have numb areas on the side of the chest and in the leg – where the arteries and veins were removed.
> - Nightmares are very common in the first few weeks.
> - Memory isn't quite what it used to be.
>
> Be assured these feelings are temporary and you'll soon be back to normal.

Valve surgery

Sometimes narrowed valves can be repaired, but in most cases of narrowed or leaking valves the diseased valve is removed and replaced with either a mechanical or a tissue replacement. Your surgeon will decide which is best for you.

Mechanical valves

These can be tilting discs or leaflets, or a 'ball in a cage' variety. Because they are made of metal and modern plastics, clots can form on them, so most patients with these valves are likely to be on anticoagulant medication – usually warfarin – for life. (See Appendix A – The drugs we take, p. 95.)

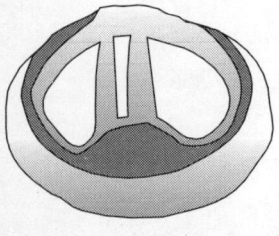

Bi-leaflet valve

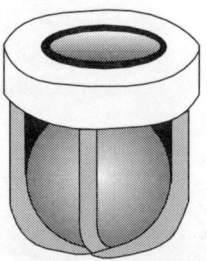

Ball and cage

Animal tissue valves

These may be valves taken from a pig's heart (which is about the same size as the human heart) or a valve fashioned from other animal tissue.

The advantage of animal tissue valves is that generally there is no need for lifelong commitment to anticoagulants. The disadvantage is that after eight–ten years such valves can deteriorate and may need replacing.

Homograft valves

A homograft valve is a human valve transplanted from a donor. These valves are similar to the animal tissue valves, but tend to last longer. The supply, however, is limited.

Percutaneous balloon valvuloplasty

Sometimes a narrowed valve (especially the mitral valve) can be opened with a technique similar to angioplasty (see p. 38). A catheter with a small balloon attached to its end is inserted through an artery in the leg to the heart, where it is inserted into the narrowed valve and the balloon inflated.

Surgery for heart failure

If heart failure cannot be controlled with medication, sometimes surgical procedures may be needed. For example, coronary artery bypass graft (CABG) (see p. 40) or angioplasty (see p. 38) may be used to treat heart failure caused by blocked arteries. Or if the underlying cause is a damaged valve, its repair or replacement may be what will be recommended.

However, if the heart is severely damaged and has only limited efficiency, the best option may be heart transplant.

Heart transplant

Since the first human heart transplant in 1967 the procedure has developed to where nowadays recipients can, with the help of modern medication, live long and fulfilled lives. Unfortunately, there are far more prospective recipients than donors, so allocation criteria are strict and tend to favour the younger patients who will benefit most from the transplant.

> **Being an organ donor**
>
> If you wish to donate any of your organs you should first of all make your wishes known to your family. You can also make a note of it in your will; but the important people to tell are your next of kin.
>
> When discussing it with your family see if any other members would also like it to be known that they are happy to donate their organs to benefit someone else.
>
> It can often ease the grieving process knowing that your loss is helping someone else; many strong bonds have been made between the families of givers and receivers.

The future

Over recent years cardiologists have been looking at both new surgical procedures and various mechanical devices that will assist the heart. These are still in the experimental stage, although it is thought that we are not too far away from developing new means to ease the suffering of those who have severe heart failure. There are also developments in introducing new muscle cells to replace damaged ones, and encouraging the heart to grow new blood vessels. It will not be too long before many of today's operations will be a thing of the past.

Some gifted people we've lost to heart disease

Gustav Mahler	Matthew Arnold
Henry Miller	Benny Goodman
Pieter Paul Rubens	Sir Alexander Fleming
Paul Gauguin	Orson Welles
Dmitri Shostakovich	Robert Browning
Mark Twain	William Butler Yeats
Sir Arthur Conan Doyle	Carl Gustav Jung

And they got through to a pretty good age without the benefits of modern techniques and medicines. So imagine what you can achieve with some exercise and a change in diet. It's worth a thought ...

4
Beating the odds – recovery, rehabilitation and prevention

> Happy are they that hear their detractions, and can put them to mending.
>
> William Shakespeare, *Much Ado About Nothing* (1598–99)

There comes a time where you're over the initial shock of being told that perhaps all is not well with the ticker and you're ready to begin living the rest of your life. And really, it's not that frightening is it? Not nowadays when there's so much that the doctors can do with medicines and the new technology.

You've learned about the heart and some of the things that can go wrong with it. Your doctor or your hospital have given you a whole pile of information on how you can improve your diet; you've been told that the body needs exercise and you've been warned of the dangers of smoking. Everyone's done their bit and now it's up to you.

So where do you start? Let's first look at exactly what has to be done.

The road to recovery

This is not as difficult a journey as you may think and at the end of it is the reward of a healthy body, a happy mind and, we believe, a more satisfying and fulfilling lifestyle. And we're not just talking about the patient – take this road and it will positively affect your family, your friends ... your whole life.

Why do we believe this? Quite simply, it's because what we're suggesting isn't just good for the health of your heart, it's good for your whole body. We've seen it time and time again.

- Learn about your heart and you'll begin to appreciate your whole body.
- Appreciate your body and you'll have no trouble getting that diet just right.
- Get the diet right and you'll begin to want to exercise.

- Exercise and you'll find it relaxes you.
- Relax and you'll laugh a lot more.
- And aren't those who laugh the happy ones?

The 'Let's Get Healthy' plan

Learn a little
Get to understand your heart and what the problem with it is. You'll find that understanding the cause will make it much easier to make the lifestyle changes necessary to get you back to good health.

Eat healthy food
Look at your diet and change it so that you're getting more of the food that's good for you and less of what's bad. Don't rush madly into it; take your time, learn what's good and what's bad, and you'll be pleasantly surprised at just how tasty a good, balanced diet can be and how well it can make you feel. (See We are what we eat, p. 54.) Also, give some thought to supplementation; because of the lack of nutrients needed in our food many people consider it important to take additional antioxidants and minerals. (See Dietary supplements, p. 92.)

Get more exercise
Remember that old saying 'Look after the body and the mind will look after itself.' It's not just the mind that will be looked after; also, more than any other organ in your body, it will bring new life to your heart. You don't have to run marathons – 30 minutes a day is plenty. (See Keeping the body moving, p. 70.)

Be more relaxed
As you get your diet right and you exercise regularly you won't find it too difficult to be more relaxed. (See Coping with stress, p. 75.)

Laugh a lot
It may not be the best medicine in the world but it certainly helps.

Give up smoking
If you are still puffing away, give it up – it really is a killer and will undo all the other good work you do. There are a lot of people out there who will help you. (See Appendix C – Useful addresses, p. 105.)

BEATING THE ODDS
Cardiac rehabilitation

Cardiac rehabilitation is the process of recovering and learning how to live with a heart condition. There are many different types of rehabilitation programmes, run either in conjunction with local hospitals or by local independent community groups. Their aim is to help individuals understand their condition and take the necessary steps towards recovery.

Your doctor should be able to direct you to a rehabilitation programme in your area but if you need further information contact the British Heart Foundation (see Appendix C – Useful addresses, p. 105).

Why do you need rehabilitation?

Studies throughout the world have shown that individuals who have been through a structured rehabilitation programme are less likely to have further problems from their heart condition, and in many cases may even reduce their need for medication.

The same research has also shown that those who go through a rehabilitation programme and stay with the changes they have made find a whole new lease of life and become, in themselves and in their families, happier, more contented people. Rehabilitation works!

What does a rehabilitation programme consist of?

Programmes differ greatly, but generally they will be made up of the following elements:

- *Education* Talks on risk factors, how to minimize the risks, diet and nutrition, the value of exercise, the drugs you take, how to manage stress, and various other matters that are relevant to your heart health.
- *Physical exercise* Monitored by healthcare professionals, you will be taken through a series of exercises so that you learn to know your own capabilities. Such a programme will cover duration and intensity of exercise and will progress to the level where you feel most comfortable.
- *Ongoing programmes and support* Rehabilitation must be ongoing, and to encourage people to continue with the good work that they started on the programme, many groups will steer people

towards healthy physical activities such as exercise and swimming classes, group walks, dancing, meditation, t'ai chi, etc.
- *Access to counselling* Many people with heart disease find it difficult to cope, and most rehabilitation groups will have access to psychological and emotional support.

Forms of rehabilitation

If you have a family history of heart problems and you've been experiencing chest pains (angina), it's not so much rehabilitation that's needed as an education programme to help you to understand the problem and how you can best combat and reverse it. There are many 'support' groups around so don't be shy – discuss it with your doctor.

If you have a heart attack and find yourself in hospital, you are likely to be offered a more formal rehabilitation programme that starts after you have been discharged. Members of the rehabilitation team will visit you while you're in hospital, explain the programme and encourage you to take part in it.

If you have surgery the rehabilitation programme may start more gently, but the messages tend to be the same.

There are three phases of rehabilitation:

- *Phase 1* takes place in hospital, where the rehabilitation team will begin to counsel you on your condition and on how you can best manage it. Topics discussed will be nutrition, the importance of exercise, the need to stop smoking and other matters related to modifying your lifestyle.
- *Phase 2* starts after you leave hospital and will vary according to local conditions. In general, programmes are run over 10 to 12 weeks, during which time your exercise levels will be monitored and your fitness levels improved. There may also be a series of educational talks for you and members of your family.
- *Phase 3* is often called the 'maintenance' phase. This is when you bring together all you've learned and continue to eat a balanced diet, have regular exercise, and together with your family learn to take life a little easier, laugh a lot and be happy.

Most rehabilitation groups are kept small so that attention can be given to the individual. Courses will last anywhere from 4 to 12 weeks.

BEATING THE ODDS
Prevention

(Refer also to the section on Risk factors, p. 25, and Chapter 5.) This is for people who have not had an event – yet!

As we learn more about heart disease it becomes quite clear that it is a disease that we can do much to anticipate and prevent. Any of us can identify with the risk factors (see So who's at risk? p. 24) and it doesn't take a nuclear scientist to work out if we should or shouldn't be concerned. As we get older and closer to the 'dangerous years' it becomes critical for us to realize how much we are at risk and what preventative action we need to take.

If you are concerned, your starting point should be your doctor, who will arrange for you to have the appropriate preventative tests (see What the doctors can do, p. 31).

> **Calcium scoring**
>
> This is a test that can make a huge difference to people with heart disease. A simple, painless CT scan with one of the new generation of ultrafast scanners enables doctors to see calcium in the coronary arteries. As the only arteries that contain calcium are the arteries that contain plaque, the build-up can be detected before it causes any symptoms.
>
> Early recognition of heart disease enables both you and your doctor to look at changes that will slow or even reverse the disease.

Many commercial companies run heart awareness programmes for their staff and some of the more enlightened ones hold educational classes and have health assessments for their more senior personnel.

It has been said that prevention can be likened to getting a head start on rehabilitation: you have the same challenges – education, exercise and nutrition – but you're not coming from behind. As the old saying goes, 'Prevention is better than cure.' We'd add three more words to that ... 'and it's easier'!

The role of the family

In writing this book our attention has mainly been focused on individuals who may be at risk of heart disease or those who have perhaps already been diagnosed with the condition.

However, heart disease is unlike a cold that will simply run its course over a few days and then be gone. It is something that is going to have a long-term effect not only on the sufferer but also on the whole family household. It is important for everyone to understand that they have a significant role to play in helping their loved one make the necessary changes so that life can continue even better than before.

And we say advisedly, 'even better than before', because the changes necessary for a healthy heart will also lead to the whole family enjoying a more satisfactory and fulfilling lifestyle.

So how can the family help?

- First and foremost, get to understand what the problem is and why changes need to be made.
- Be patient – after a heart event, many people lose confidence, tire easily, suffer unaccustomed depression and get somewhat snappy. It is a temporary condition and rest assured it doesn't last. (See Depression, p. 81.)
- It's important to realize that your patient (for lack of another phrase) is most probably very scared and trying very hard to keep it from the rest of the family. This particularly applies to the male of the species who seems to think that he should have a macho attitude in front of everyone! Try and explain that in sharing one's worries or concerns, they really do become much lighter to carry. (See Chapter 6.)
- Offer encouragement and support whenever you can – let them know they are not alone and be there with them on doctor or hospital visits.
- It's not a good idea to treat your patient as if they're made of cut glass. They are unlikely to be in danger and the sooner they are up and about, the sooner you will all get your lives back to a semblance of normality.
- If your patient finds going for walks quite boring, why not help them out and set up a rota among the family so they are never out alone. (See Keeping the body moving, p. 70.)
- If a diet change is called for, why not apply it to the whole family – food that's healthy for the heart is healthy for the whole body and everyone will be a winner. And think of the fun you can all have exploring some of the new heart healthy cookbooks that are now available. (See We are what we eat, p. 54, and Appendix B, Suggested reading, p. 103.)
- Any smokers in the family, particularly your patient, should be encouraged to stop. It really is a killer and will have an effect on everyone in the household! (See Smoking, p. 28.)

- The chances are that your patient will be on some form of medication. Learn what the medicines are for and help make sure that they are taken as directed. (See Medication, p. 37, and Appendix A, The drugs we take, p. 95.)
- No matter how beneficial changes will be in the long term, in the short term they are going to cause some stress. Discuss things as a whole family before any changes are made. (See Coping with stress, p. 75.)
- We all need a treat now and again so don't be too rigorous with the rules and give yourselves one now and again – it'll do you the world of good.

One final point. When a family works together in support of the health of one of its members, one of the outcomes is that young members of the family learn at an early age the benefits of a good, healthy lifestyle and are likely to build their own lives, and the lives of their children, accordingly.

Getting started

If you've looked at the risk factors for heart disease and feel that perhaps it's time for you to take some preventative measures, may we recommend the following. Go to the beginning of this section, study what we've called the 'Let's Get Healthy' plan (p. 46), and together with your family work out a strategy that best suits you. Here are a few hints to get you on your way.

First, think about your diet. (See We are what we eat, p. 54.)

- Remember there's nothing that you can't eat – it's just that you should eat a little less of some of the things you might like – but which don't like you.
- You'll be surprised at the tasty things you can do with those foods you're not so keen on – we've listed a few cookbooks that have a lot of great suggestions for good, healthy, easy-to-make recipes.
- Think balance and trade-off; yes, on a hot summer's day treat yourself to an ice cream (only one though!) – but then balance that over the next few days with extra helpings of those good-for-you dark green or coloured vegetables or fruit.
- Think alternatives. Instead of crisps or biscuits for that afternoon snack, why not try some dried fruit? And have you ever noticed the large range of nuts that supermarkets carry nowadays? (But

it's best to roast them yourself – commercial producers use the cheap fats which are bad.)
- Be a bit adventurous – think salsas, chillies and mustards. There's a whole new world out there.
- Take a look at the Mediterranean diet (see p. 57) – olive oil, fish, fruit, legumes, breads, red wine. It sounds yummy – and it is – and your heart will bless you.

Now what about exercise? (See Keeping the body moving, p. 70.)
Your body is not as hard a taskmaster as you may think – just like any piece of sophisticated engineering, all it asks is to be kept in good running order.

- If you can add up your exercise time to around 30 or 40 minutes every day, that should keep you in fairly good shape; though the more you do the better you'll feel.
- How do you squeeze 30 minutes of exercise into an already busy day? Here are some suggestions.
  - Walk or take the bus to work instead of driving.
  - When you take the bus, walk an extra stop or two at either end of your journey.
  - Ignore lifts and walk. (If you're on the sixteenth floor take the lift to the twelfth and walk the rest of the way.) Always walk down.
  - Get a few friends together and go dancing – amazing how much exercise you get out of a Latin American medley!
  - On a wet day, park at a shopping centre and do a little bit of fast window-shopping.
- Buy a good book on exercising.

Stop smoking

We can't stress this strongly enough. Here's what you gain by quitting:

- reduced risk of heart disease
- reduced risk of emphysema
- reduced risk of lung cancer. In fact, smoking causes cancer in every tissue it touches – tongue, larynx, lung, stomach and bladder – to name but a few!
- increased lifespan
- improved quality of life – and you don't smell!
- whiter teeth and fresher breath
- no nagging cough.

BEATING THE ODDS

The silver lining *Most people who have a heart event and make the necessary changes in their lifestyle report that the quality of their life improves dramatically. Their relationship with their spouse becomes stronger, and they have a healthier self-image, a better ability to handle work pressures, and a whole new enthusiasm for the simple pleasures in life.*

5
Living with heart disease

Of all human foibles love of living is the most powerful.
> Molière, *Love's the Best Doctor* (1665)

This is the part of the book that all three of us – doctor, patient and cardiologist – find the most exciting. Although we know that heart disease is increasing at an alarming rate and that it is affecting people at a younger age, we are also learning that not only is the disease controllable, but in many cases it is also reversible.

And this gives us hope – that with this knowledge we, as a society, will be able to diagnose those at risk of heart disease much earlier than we do at present; that with the understanding that we can control our heart disease through lifestyle changes, more of us will make the effort to do so; and finally, the hope that we will teach our children the value of a considered healthy lifestyle, so they don't repeat our errors.

This part of the book is dedicated to that hope.

We are what we eat

In this section we will look at the effects certain foods have on our body and how an appropriate diet can reduce the risk of developing heart disease. We understand that most of us don't relish the thought of changing the habits of a lifetime, so before you throw your hands in the air in frustration, may we offer you the following incentives.

- Get the right balance in the food you eat and you will greatly reduce your risk of developing heart disease.
- If you already have heart disease, a balanced diet – coupled with exercise – will help to hold it in check or, in many cases, reverse it.
- You will certainly lose some weight.
- You'll feel much better. After a while, most people who change to a healthier diet wish they had done so much earlier.
- It's not really as difficult as you may think.
- And the good thing about making a change to some of the new

foods and recipes that are available is that they are actually healthy. (See Appendix B – Suggested reading, p. 103.)

> **Eating's a family affair**
>
> Most people live in a family with their partner and their children and it is unlikely that more than one person in that family will have a heart condition.
>
> *Question* Should all the family adhere to the diet regime?
> *Answer* Yes, *yes*, **yes**!
>
> Eating a healthy balanced diet shouldn't be just for those with a heart condition – it should be for everybody. Of course, younger children have different needs and you must make allowances for these, but in general you will be doing them a favour by instilling in them good eating habits. Remember, you probably laid down the foundation for your heart disease in your teens.
>
> Also, as a family you will not be isolating the patient among you; quite the reverse, you will be showing them how much you all care.

So what is a healthy diet?

A healthy diet – and not just for good heart health, but for the whole body – is first and foremost a matter of balance of the proteins, carbohydrates, minerals and vitamins that our bodies need. Get that balance right and you'll be well on the way to having not only a healthy heart and body, but also a very healthy and happy mind.

Of course, there are some foods you should eat and plenty that you shouldn't – or only have a little of – but no one is going to regiment their lives to the extent of only eating what's good for them and never touching those things that are perhaps not so good. You compromise a little, trade off here and there and find a balance you can live with. It all comes down to how much you care!

Changing your diet *It's an interesting fact that when people change to a healthy heart diet they suddenly find themselves eating a much wider range of food than they did before – and enjoying it more!*

The foods your body needs

Carbohydrates
Carbohydrates, starches and sugars, provide the fuel we need to run our bodies.

Carbohydrates are found in vegetables, fruit, rice, cereals and sugars – and not just breakfast cereals but all products made from flour, such as bread and pasta.

Proteins
Proteins are found throughout the body in muscles, tendons, skin, blood and, of course, as the base material of our bones. Not only does protein help our bodies grow, but also in later life it helps us cope with the wear and tear of living. Dietary protein, that which we eat, is a source of the amino acids our body needs to make its own protein.

Proteins are found in meat, poultry, fish, dairy products (not butter), eggs, tofu (soy bean curd), beans, wholegrain cereals and lentils.

Minerals
Most of us are aware that minerals are needed for our bones and teeth, but they also have many other important functions that keep our bodies working.

Some of the more common minerals used by our body are calcium, iron, magnesium, potassium, sodium and zinc.

Vitamins
Vitamins are essential for the body to work efficiently. The word comes from VITal AMINes. Our body cannot make these, so they must come from our food.

The vitamins for a healthy heart are A, B-complex, C, D, E and K. (See Dietary supplements, p. 92.)

Fats
Fats, as well as being important building blocks for the cells of our bodies, are also the most efficient way we can consume and store energy. There are some essential fats which our bodies can't make, so we must get them from the food we eat. Examples of these are the omega-3 fatty acid, found in fish, and some vegetable oils, both of which are particularly good for the heart.

LIVING WITH HEART DISEASE
The foods that are good for us

Carbohydrates
Vegetables, fruit, beans and whole-grain foods (complex carbohydrates) are at the very core of healthy eating. They are packed with fibre, minerals and naturally occurring antioxidants, and have clearly shown that they contribute greatly to lowering the risk of heart disease – and as an extra bonus they are also protective against some cancers.

Vegetables
Freshly picked vegetables are rich in minerals, B vitamins, vitamin C, fibre and antioxidants. Lightly boiled or steamed, microwaved, stir-fried in a little olive oil or eaten raw, they are very, very good for you. The greener the better – so go for broccoli, cabbage, spinach, courgettes, peas, French beans and lettuces. And, of course, avocados – they're a healthy type of fat and a great source of vitamin E.

Don't forget the other coloured vegetables: carrots, pumpkins, aubergines, red, green and yellow peppers, onions, etc.

If you boil your vegetables, why not use the water when making soup?

Frozen vegetables are OK, but don't overcook them; just put a little water in the bottom of the pan and steam them with the lid on.

Try this!

How about a 'warm salad'? Stir-fry – in a little olive oil – sliced onions, cubes of carrot and other root vegetables and lay them over a bed of diced raw vegetables – for example, a mix of lettuces, tomato, cucumber, avocado and grated carrot. To top it off, sprinkle with cashew nuts.

Now and again you could also stir-fry in some chicken or lean pork – but not too much! Or what about adding a small tin of tuna? The possibilities are endless.

If you're eating out, a warm salad is a pretty safe bet and it could give you some ideas for what you could do yourself at home.

The Mediterranean diet
Not so much a diet but rather an approach to life, the Mediterranean diet came to prominence when it was realized that people living in

countries around the Mediterranean Sea – particularly Italy, Greece, France, and Spain – had an extremely low incidence of heart disease. So what *is* their secret?

Simple: a cuisine low in saturated fat and red meat, and high in fish and plant products such as vegetables, fruit, pasta, grains, beans, olives and olive oil – all accompanied by a glass or two of red wine. Put that together with a relaxed lifestyle and it seems you've got a recipe for a pretty healthy way of life.

There are many books that give information and recipes on the Mediterranean diet.

Fruit

Remember that old saying, 'An apple a day keeps the doctor away'? Nowadays it's not just apples that keep the doctor at bay, but all fruit, such as apples, oranges, peaches, pears, all berries, all melons, bananas, grapefruit and all those exotic tropical fruits we now have in our supermarkets.

Dried fruit is high in fibre and potassium and has some iron. On the other hand, vitamin C is lost in the drying process and dried fruit can be loaded with concentrated sugar.

Tinned fruit will also serve you well, but only that canned in juice – not syrup, as syrup contains a large amount of sugar.

Many fresh fruit juices contain vitamin C and other goodies, but can also be very high in sugar.

Try this!

The old classic with a new twist – *fresh* fruit salad.

Cut, peel and chop a mix of all the fresh fruit in season and add a little white wine and/or fruit juice to stop it going brown. You may also like to add some fresh, frozen or tinned blue- or blackberries. Top it off with a sprinkling of plain or roasted sliced almonds. Serve with yoghurt or custard made with low-fat milk.

Garlic

This may not be everyone's cup of tea but it's been around since the Middle Ages as a natural medicine. Garlic contains potassium, B and C vitamins, as well as some calcium, and does a wonderful job of making the blood less sticky and thus reducing its tendency to clot. Some doctors do not support its use because there is little evidence that garlic does good; there is also no evidence it does harm. There is just no evidence – yet.

You can take garlic as a supplement, which won't leave an unpleasant odour on your breath (see Dietary supplements, p. 92).

Try this!
Take a few peeled garlic cloves, crush them into a paste with a little salt, fry lightly in a pan with olive oil and add chopped onions, fresh parsley, basil, tarragon – or any combination of herbs you fancy. Immediately add chopped mushrooms and tomatoes for just a couple of minutes and then pile onto a slice of wholegrain bread. Garnish with a little feta cheese and olives.

Flavonoids

These are a powerful group of antioxidants, found in a wide variety of fruits and vegetables: apples, onions and green beans are particularly flavonoid-rich, as are black and green tea.

Red wine – in moderation – is considered good for the heart because it is made from red grapes which are high in flavonoids. (See Alcohol, page 64.)

Antioxidants stop the action of free radicals, which are a major cause of many diseases including coronary artery disease, stroke, cancer, arthritis, diabetes, Alzheimer's, osteoporosis – to name but a few. (See Antioxidants, page 65.)

Wholegrains

Wheat, rice, oats, corn, barley and buckwheat are the most common wholegrain foods. These contain many vitamins and are rich in health-preserving fibre.

As wholegrains lose much of their nutrients in milling, particularly the B vitamins and vitamin E, try to eat them whenever possible as unmilled wholegrains.

> **Try this!**
>
> Here's a good way to start the day.
>
> In a bowl, mix 1/3 cup of oatmeal with about 1/2 cup of water (depending on how you like it) and slip it into the microwave for 2–3 minutes. Top with sliced fresh fruit and a little natural yoghurt – unsweetened so you can add your own brown sugar. You may also like to add a sprinkling of sunflower and pumpkin seeds, pine nuts, etc. If you like your porridge a little more milky, just add some low-fat milk.

Don't forget about that great Italian stand-by – pasta. It comes in many shapes and sizes with equally as many types of sauces to choose from. But do be careful about the sauces, as some can be seriously loaded with the bad fats.

Beans

Low in fat and rich in protein, complex carbohydrates and fibre – of the kind that is especially good for lowering blood cholesterol – beans should be an essential part of your diet. Dried beans are best soaked overnight, but the tinned variety are OK and very convenient. Check out your supermarket shelves – they have a comprehensive variety.

> **Try this!**
>
> Here's a great northern Spanish dish for those cold winter nights.
>
> Soak overnight a mix of your favourite beans – kidney beans, broad beans, red and brown beans, chick-peas – whatever you fancy. Next day drain and cover well with a vegetable soup stock. Add seasoning, crushed garlic and some chilli peppers to taste, then cook until the beans are tender (about an hour). Heat and serve with large chunks of black bread.
>
> Now and again it wouldn't hurt if you also added a small amount of sliced salami – but very little, just to add taste.

Proteins

For most of us our main source of protein has traditionally come from eating meat, dairy products or eggs. So quite naturally, when we look at reducing the risk of heart disease one of the first things we consider doing is to cut back on these foods. However, this is perhaps not such a good idea as they are an important source of other nutrients we need in our diet – such as iron, zinc and B complex vitamins.

If we cut back too much on proteins we run the risk of becoming 'protein deficient' which in turn can lead to a loss of muscle mass (especially in those who are less active physically); this could result in increased body fat and higher cholesterol levels.

Alternatives to meat and dairy products are:

Fish

From the point of view of the heart – fish is it! It contains a type of fatty acid called omega-3, which has many beneficial qualities, in particular the ability to raise the level of good cholesterol (HDL) in our blood. Diets high in fish also have a stabilizing effect on the heart rhythm and people with a high fish diet have fewer cardiac arrests when they have a heart attack than non-fish lovers. But do watch out for those rich batters and sauces!

Shellfish not only taste good but are highly nutritious as well. In the past people were told that shellfish had high cholesterol levels, but now, because we know of their omega-3 content, it's accepted that they are fine eaten in modest amounts – probably the best news of the decade for shellfish lovers!

Tinned fish will give you all the proteins and minerals of fresh fish, although it may not retain all its omega-3 fatty acids or vitamins.

Flaxseed (linseed)

Flaxseed is high in omega-3 oils. When ground, flaxseed can be added to bread recipes, sprinkled on hot or cold cereals or stirred into fruit or vegetable juice. It can be used to supplement your fish diet.

- Flaxseed oil is excellent in salad dressings or poured over vegetables.
- There is not much point in eating the seeds whole, as the body won't digest them.
- Flaxseed oil is also available in capsule form as a supplement.

Soy foods

If you're looking for a meat substitute you can't go far wrong with soy. It provides protein and antioxidants, and will help lower your bad cholesterol and raise the good.

Tofu, also called soybean curd or bean curd, is made as an extract from cooked soybeans. Rich in protein, calcium and iron, it is an ideal meat substitute and can be used in casseroles, stir-fries, salads, sandwiches or soup.

Tempeh, made by fermenting soybeans which are then pressed into a cake, is an excellent meat substitute in stir-fries.

Miso, rich in B vitamins and protein, can be used in soups, sauces, dips and marinades.

Soy milk (fortified), which has no saturated fat, can be used whenever a recipe calls for cow's milk.

Minerals

(See Dietary supplements, p. 92.)

The most common minerals that affect our heart are calcium, magnesium, potassium and sodium. If you're eating a mixed, balanced diet you should be getting the minerals you need – although if you're 'salt sensitive' you ought to keep an eye on your sodium intake.

Calcium

The most abundant mineral in our body is calcium; in addition to keeping our bones strong, it helps the heart to beat regularly. Calcium deficiency rarely affects the heart, but it does affect our bones.

Calcium mainly comes from milk and milk products such as yoghurt and cheese; other good sources are dark green vegetables, salmon and sardines, soybeans, dried beans, peanuts and walnuts.

Magnesium

This promotes a healthy cardiovascular system and helps prevent rhythm disorders, especially after heart attacks. It also helps us relax and sleep better.

The best natural sources of magnesium are dark green vegetables, lemons, grapefruit, figs, sweetcorn, almonds, nuts, seeds.

Potassium

Potassium is essential for stable heart function. If the blood levels of this mineral become low – especially common when diuretics (fluid-draining pills) are being used – heart rhythm disturbances can occur. If you're on this type of medication your doctor may prescribe a potassium supplement.

If potassium levels are too high, you might experience heart rhythm disturbances.

You'll find potassium in potatoes, citrus fruits, bananas, leafy green vegetables, watercress, sunflower seeds and mint leaves.

Sodium

Sodium is a mineral to be wary of: too much salt in your diet can promote high blood pressure, especially if you are 'salt sensitive'. You need some, but not too much.

Don't add salt while cooking – flavour to taste at the table and use 'natural' or 'sea' salt which contains minerals other than sodium chloride (common table salt). Other options are herbs and spices – but beware of monosodium glutamate (MSG).

Sodium is found in abundance in most processed, convenience food. Particularly watch out for salted cured meats such as ham, bacon and corned beef, condiments such as soy and chilli sauces and ketchup, and spreads such as Marmite and Bovril. Beware also of hidden salt in tinned vegetables and food from your local takeaway.

Vitamins

(See Dietary supplements, p. 92.)

Vitamins are organic substances essential for life which cannot be made or synthesized by our bodies. In their natural state they are found in natural foods – and that's the best source to get them from.

Our heart, as well as the rest of our body, benefits from all the vitamins, in particular the following:

Vitamin A

One of the nutrients essential for healing wounds after surgery, vitamin A also helps to ward off infections.

Foods high in vitamin A (or its precursors, carotenes) include sweet potatoes, carrots, pumpkin, spinach, courgettes, tomatoes, rock melons and evaporated skimmed milk.

Vitamin B6, B12 and folic acid

Low levels of these vitamins can increase the risk of coronary artery disease because they raise the level in the blood of a toxic compound called homocysteine (See p. 26.)

The best sources of these are:

- B6: cabbage, wheat bran, wheatgerm, wholegrain bread, brewer's yeast, cantaloupe melons, eggs, beef, milk, liver, kidney.

- B12: beef, pork, kidney, liver, cheese, eggs, milk.
- Folic acid: deep green vegetables, carrots, avocados, beans, pumpkins, whole wheat, wholegrains, melon, apricots, egg yolk, liver.

Vitamin C (a powerful antioxidant)
As well as helping to decrease cholesterol levels, vitamin C also accelerates healing after surgery, lowers the incidence of blood clots and generally helps our body live a long and healthy life. Some people also swear they get fewer colds – though trials show this is perhaps wishful thinking!

The best natural sources are freshly picked citrus fruits, berries, green leafy vegetables, cauliflower, tomatoes, potatoes and sweet potatoes.

Note Vitamin C levels fall when fruit is stored.

Vitamin E
An all-round vitamin, it helps prevent and dissolve blood clots, lowers blood pressure and when applied externally will help prevent the formation of scar tissue. Both vitamins C and E are powerful antioxidants, and in preventing heart disease they work well together.

Sources of vitamin E are vegetable oils (particularly cold-pressed virgin olive oil) and products made with them, wheatgerm, wholegrains, nuts and seeds.

Liquids

Our bodies need liquid. Unfortunately nowadays when we get thirsty we tend to reach for a drink that contains sugar, caffeine or fat. Next time your body calls out for some liquid why not give it some good old-fashioned water? Or you could try one of the many mineral waters that are now on the market, though beware of 'sports' drinks – they contain large amounts of caffeine.

Tea – black or green (though not herbal) – is also good for you as it is high in flavonoids (see Flavonoids, p. 59).

Alcohol
Although there are many conflicting opinions regarding alcohol and the heart, what everyone does agree on is that a glass or two of your favourite wine with a meal each day may lower the risk of heart disease. If your choice is red wine you will also get some antioxidant benefit.

But if you drink more than that – or more than one or two beers, or more than two standard measures of spirits a day – then the chances are you'll be raising your blood pressure and therefore adding to the risk. In large doses alcohol can poison your heart, so keep it down to those two small glasses per day.

Antioxidants, free radicals and oxidation

Free radicals are a toxic by-product produced as our bodies use oxygen. They have a mind of their own and like loose cannons they run riot through our bloodstream, damaging cells in general and our LDL cholesterol particles in particular.

These damaged particles swell in the artery walls and kill nearby cells; many believe this is the major cause of plaque and the narrowing of the arteries. It is also the oxidized LDL in the plaque that ruptures into the artery, causing a heart attack.

These little devils are also believed to contribute to ageing, cancer and other diseases, so clearly it is wise to protect against them.

The antioxidants found in fresh fruit and vegetables, and in supplements, neutralize free radicals.

There are four ways we can limit the damage done by free radicals.

- If you are using fat, use monounsaturated.
- Eat plenty of fruit and vegetables.
- Beta carotene (a form of vitamin A) and vitamins E and C are antioxidants.
- Flavonoids found in grape seeds and skins, red wine and green tea are powerful antioxidants.

What to watch out for

Fat – The Public Enemy Number One that can also be a friend

We can't live without it and – for many of us – we can't live with it. Eating the wrong dietary fat is the main cause of our having high blood cholesterol levels and this is one of the major risk factors in developing heart disease (see Cholesterol, p. 25).

Basically there are three types of fat – bad, mixed blessing and good.

Saturated fat: the baddy
This is your heart's greatest enemy. It typically comes from animal sources (the fat on meat – beef, pork, lamb, chicken) and dairy

products – though certain plant fats such as cocoa butter, palm and coconut oil are also saturated. Eating saturated fats raises your level of bad cholesterol and lowers that of the good.

Polyunsaturated fat: the mixed blessing
Neither good nor bad, polyunsaturated fat primarily comes from vegetable sources such as corn, sunflower, safflower, sesame, etc. These have no effect on cholesterol levels.

Monounsaturated fat: the goody
This most heart-friendly of fats comes from vegetable sources such as olives or olive oil. Taking these raises your good cholesterol (HDL) and lowers the bad (LDL). Cold-pressed virgin olive oil is also a great source of vitamin E.

Meat

If you're going to eat meat then here are a few hints you should take note of:

- Processed meats – unless they're labelled 'low-fat' – are generally loaded with saturated fats. Watch out for salami, sausages, hamburgers and hot dogs.
- Choose poultry rather than red meat – but avoid the skin (very fatty) and dark meat. You can't go far wrong with the white meat of a turkey.
- If you're using mince, ask for low-fat mince or mince your own lean cuts.
- Believe it or not, some hamburgers have more saturated fat than fried chicken.
- On any meat you eat, cut away all the fat you can see.
- Eat smaller portions.

Organ meats
Unfortunately for lovers of offal – liver, kidneys, brains, sweetbreads, gizzards and hearts – these are packed full of cholesterol and saturated fats. They are very much a 'treat meat'.

For meat substitutes see Soy foods, p. 61.

Dairy products

Butter or margarine?
We know butter is loaded with saturated fat, margarine with transfatty acids. What do we do?

Fortunately we're no longer faced with this dilemma – there are now spreads which are positively beneficial. Olive oil spreads and those that have been enriched with plant sterols and stanols will actually lower your blood cholesterol levels. Sterols/stanols are naturally occurring components of all plants. They are mainly found in vegetable oils, but traces are also present in fruit and vegetables.

Cheese, cream and milk
All are high in saturated fats. Hard cheeses aren't as dangerous as soft; low-fat milk is OK; ice cream, unless it's labelled low-fat, should be on your 'only as a treat' list. Yoghurt is great for you.

Chocolate
Not only is chocolate made with full-fat milk but it also contains cocoa butter, which is one of the plant sources of saturated fat. Do not be fooled by the articles saying that chocolate contains phenols which may reduce heart disease. No chocolate-eating society has low heart attack rates. Chocolate is a definite for your 'treat' list.

Cocoa powder, on the other hand, can be used in cooking to add flavour because much of the cocoa butter has been removed in its manufacture.

Eggs
These used to be considered as pure poison, but are now thought to be not so bad. If you have high cholesterol don't eat more than two or three eggs a week (any way but fried) – otherwise they are fine in moderation.

The villain of the egg is the yolk, so if you're partial to omelettes or scrambled eggs, use one whole egg and one white instead of two whole. You might also consider a similar technique in any recipe that doesn't require too many eggs.

And beware of quiche – it can hide some pretty heart-unhealthy fat!

Sodium *(common table salt)*
The main problem with sodium is that it causes high blood pressure. If you tend to have high blood pressure or have heart failure, it is important that you are aware of your salt intake.

Beware of convenience, processed, tinned and fast foods – they generally contain high levels of sodium.

> **Trans-fatty acids and hydrogenation**
> Hydrogenation is the process used in making shortening and margarine, whereby liquid vegetable oils are converted to solid or semi-solid trans-fatty acids.
>
> Though derived from good vegetable oils, trans-fatty acids act more like saturated fat in that they increase the levels of bad cholesterol (LDL) and reduce the good (HDL).
>
> Monounsaturated oils – rapeseed and peanut – convert into trans-fatty acids with heating, so it's best to use olive oil for cooking.
>
> Because trans-fatty acids increase the shelf-life of commercially prepared foods, they will be found in many processed convenience foods such as potato crisps, biscuits, cake mixes and frozen foods.
>
> Treat trans-fatty acids as if they were saturated fats – they are *baddies*.

Bread and biscuits

No bread is really bad for you – unless you load it with butter or margarine! – but change from white bread to wholemeal, wholegrain or rye loaves. Supermarkets nowadays carry a great selection to choose from.

Beware of croissants – basically they're bread with lots of extra fat added before they are baked.

Try baking your own bread and loading it with nuts and seeds. Even with modern bread-baking machines it gives a real sense of achievement, smells fabulous and is good for you.

Those sweet biscuits that we like with our tea or coffee are generally loaded with saturated fat and sugar. Try crackers or crispbread with one of the excellent low-fat dips that are now available. Beware of potato crisps – they are full of saturated fat.

Sugar

As far as the heart is concerned a little sugar won't do you any damage: the problem is the excess sugar we may have in our bodies. With the high amounts of sugar hiding in processed, convenience foods, many of us quite unwittingly eat far more than we should. Our bodies turn any excess sugar or alcohol into triglycerides and other fats, and high levels of these increase the risk of heart disease and weight-related problems.

Note that 'natural' sugars are not significantly different from normal sugar.

If you have a family history of the type of diabetes that shows itself in adulthood, you should be especially careful of your sugar intake and have your blood sugar levels checked regularly.

> **Your new healthy diet at a glance**
>
> We all have different preferences in the food we eat and there is no set diet that will suit everybody. So let's have an overview of the sorts of food you should be eating.
>
> *To be encouraged*
> Green or dark green vegetables, and all other vegetables.
> All fish – especially oily fish.
> All fruit; dried fruit – great as a snack.
> Beans, wholegrains, breads, legumes, pasta, soy products, rice, couscous, potato.
> Nuts and seeds – raw or home roasted.
> Olive oil – as much as you want.
> Meat only once or twice a week as a garnish to the meal.
>
> *These are OK*
> Avocados, garlic, shellfish, skimmed milk.
>
> *Go easy on these*
> Animal foods (beef, corned beef, lamb, pork and ham, chicken – especially the skin).
> Dairy products (butter, cream, ice cream, full-fat milk, cheese [apart from cottage cheese]).
> Too much salt or sugar; margarine. But remember that the low-fat versions aren't too bad in small quantities.
>
> *Not encouraged*
> Snack foods: potato crisps, chocolate, biscuits, pre-packed cakes.
>
> *Dangerous!!*
> Offal.
> Processed meats – sausages, pies, salami, hamburgers, hot dogs, etc.
> Pre-packed convenience foods that aren't labelled 'low-fat'.
>
> *We need liquids*
> Water, mineral water (flat or sparkling), fruit juice, a glass or two of red wine, red grape juice, tea, herbal tea, low-fat milk.
>
> Remember – grilling is better than frying!

Eating out

One of the great pleasures of life is to go out to a restaurant with a group of friends and celebrate someone's birthday or anniversary, catch up on what's been happening and talk about the good old days. Well, whatever you do, don't let your heart stand in the way of enjoying that simple pleasure. As long as you don't make a habit of it, it's quite OK to let your hair down now and again. If you never did you'd most probably do yourself more mischief through letting tension build up rather than indulging in some forbidden delicacies.

However, unless it's a *very* special occasion you should tread a little carefully. Here are some hints that you may find helpful.

- Don't be shy. If you see something on the menu that you're not familiar with, ask about it.
- Beware creamed soups – you're better off with stock-based ones.
- If you're having chicken, ask for the chef to remove the skin – that's where most of the fat hides!
- Ask for all sauces and dressings on the side so that you're in control of how much you add.
- If there's a salad bar watch out for creamy dressings, grated cheese and chopped eggs.
- The safest foods to order are stir-fried, grilled, roasted, poached, steamed or boiled.
- Avoid fried and mashed potatoes – have them baked, boiled or roasted.

So off you go and enjoy yourself – you've most probably deserved it. But don't make a habit of it! *Bon appetit.*

Keeping the body moving

> Though it be disfigured by many defects, to whom is his body not dear.
>
> Panchatantra, *c.* 5th century

Whether you have heart disease and want to make sure you hold it in check, or your risk factors are pretty high and you're taking a preventative view, the most important thought to keep in mind is that all the good work you do won't mean much if you don't keep it up. And this particularly applies to exercise.

Just like your motor car parked out there in the garage, your body needs to be cared for and taken out for a run every now and again. Would you leave your car sitting for a few weeks or so, unattended? Unlikely. And that's a bit of machinery that can be replaced. But think how many people leave themselves sitting around, not just for a few days or weeks, but for months and even years. Unfortunately, we are not replaceable!

So let's have a look at the 'what, why, how, where and when' of exercise and examine the benefits of this easy, simple and cheap means we have of minimizing our risk of heart disease.

What is exercise?

The simplest definition of exercise is any activity that gets your heart pumping, your lungs breathing, your muscles working and your joints flexing. So any activity that does all this for you is exercise – and the activity that does it best of all is good old-fashioned walking.

> **The definition of a game of rugby** *Thirty men in desperate need of rest being watched by thousands of people in desperate need of exercise.*

Why should we exercise?
The benefits of exercise are many, particularly for your cardiovascular system. Here are some of the good things it'll do for you:

- it increases your heart's ability to pump blood
- if you have high blood pressure it can help to lower it
- it increases good cholesterol and reduces bad
- it may decrease triglyceride levels
- it helps with weight control
- it helps reduce stress.

In the longer term, regular exercise will also offer you the following benefits:

- better capacity for exercise
- improved physical and mental abilities
- less tension and anxiety
- self-confidence and a feeling of well-being.

Mainly we're talking here about walking, because this is one activity that is for everyone, irrespective of age or sex. However if you prefer some other form of activity, you go ahead with it. All the benefits enjoyed by walking also apply to other aerobic exercises. (Any activity that increases the body's endurance by enhancing its ability to use oxygen is called aerobic.)

How to exercise

One mistake many people make is that they think of exercise as that practised by professional athletes and sportspeople: the 'no pain – no gain' school of thought.

That may or may not be true for our hardy professionals, but it certainly isn't true for anyone who's trying to manage heart disease. What you should be aiming for is a level of 'moderate intensity' – that's just enough effort so that you know that you're exerting yourself. This is also called 'perceived exertion'.

Moderate intensity

So how can you judge what's moderate intensity? What is your perceived exertion? If you're walking with someone you should be able to talk quite easily without getting out of breath and if you're on your own you should have no trouble whistling or singing to yourself. If in either case it becomes somewhat uncomfortable, then you're pushing yourself too hard and you should slow down. On the other hand, if you don't feel it's any effort at all – push just that little bit more.

For the more scientific among us, you can work out your optimum exercise rate by the formula in Evaluating your heart rate on p. 73.

If you're feeling more adventurous and would like to do your exercising in a gymnasium, make sure that it is one where the instructors are familiar with the problems faced by people with heart conditions.

Accumulating exercise

One of the many wonders of the human body is that it can 'accumulate' the short bursts of activity you give it throughout the day. These will go into your 'bank' so that three bursts of 10 minutes will give you almost the same benefit as 30 minutes spent in the gym. So take a brisk 10-minute walk on the way to and from work and find some stairs at lunchtime and – hey presto! – you've done your 30 minutes for that day.

> **Evaluating your heart rate**
>
> Here's a simple way to check if you're exercising to the right level.
>
> What you're aiming for is to get to around 60–70 per cent of your maximum heart rate. You can work this out by subtracting your age from 220 – giving you your maximum heart rate – and then take 60–70 per cent of this and you have the optimum heart rate for you to exercise at.
>
> For example, if you're 40 years old, then 220 minus 40 gives you a maximum heart rate of 180, and 60–70 per cent of this shows that your heartbeats when exercising should be between 108 and 126 beats per minute.
>
> *Note* Take your heartbeat rate from your pulse, which you'll find on the thumb side of your wrist. There's a bit of a knack to it, but you'll soon get used to it.

When to exercise?

The best time to exercise is whenever you feel most comfortable. Some people prefer the early mornings, others late afternoon, and if you look around our streets at midday you'll see many brave souls using their lunch hour to get in their day's quota.

Times when you shouldn't exercise are:

- soon after a heavy meal
- if you've been lying in the sun
- if you have a fever
- if you have unresolved unstable angina
- if you have high resting blood pressure
- if you have new or recurrent symptoms of breathlessness, palpitations, dizziness or lethargy.

Note If you haven't been exercising regularly over the past few months we would strongly advise that you talk it over with your doctor before starting.

Where to exercise?

That's an easy one to answer – anywhere that gives you pleasure! Some people prefer walking near their homes and plan a number of interesting walks they can take, depending on the mood they're in.

Others may prefer to take a trip out to the country or seaside and enjoy their walk when they get there.

One place we'd suggest you don't exercise is walking along any street that's busy with motor traffic – it's unpleasant and it isn't very good for your lungs. So if the city is where you do your exercise, try to choose streets that have little or no traffic.

Think of what parks there are in your area – chances are you've driven past them many times without even noticing.

Many towns and cities have walking groups and your local council most probably has them listed.

If you're a water lover then maybe you'd like to try aqua jogging – it's an excellent way to get exercise and not put too much pressure on your joints or muscles. Perhaps your local swimming pool has aqua jogging classes.

Don't be a couch potato *The British Heart Foundation reports that people who do not exercise are twice as likely to develop coronary artery disease as those who exercise on a regular basis. If people who exercise suffer a heart attack, their risk of dying from it is half that of those who do not exercise.*

Exercise and medication

- *Beta blockers and calcium-channel blockers* Because these lower your heart rate response to exercise, you should judge the intensity of your exercise by perceived exertion rather than evaluated heart rate.
- *Diuretics* If you're taking a diuretic make sure you drink plenty of liquid before, during and after the activity.

Danger signs

If any of the following symptoms show themselves while you're exercising, stop immediately, and talk it over with your doctor before resuming any form of physical activity:

- any sort of discomfort in your chest, upper body, neck, arms or jaw
- more than normal shortness of breath
- lightheadedness or dizziness
- any change in normally felt symptoms
- your pulse skips or races.

A few hints to make life easy

- If you haven't exercised for a while, check with your doctor.
- Make sure you have comfortable shoes and loose-fitting clothes.
- Having a dog to be responsible for can make walking a pleasure.
- If you use glyceryl trinitrate spray or tablets, take one before you head out and make sure you have your spray with you.
- If you get angina pain while walking, stop and rest, then carry on – you'll find that you'll progressively walk longer distances.
- Dancing is excellent exercise and can be a lot of fun.
- T'ai chi and yoga will give you good exercise as well as helping to relieve stress.
- Keep in mind that movement can also be exercise – e.g. get up and switch off the TV rather than using the remote control. Every little helps.
- Aqua jogging is excellent for the heart and is a wonderful way of exercising if you have arthritis or are overweight.

(Also see Prevention and Getting started, pp. 49 and 52.)

Coping with stress

> What is this life if, full of care
> We have no time to stand and stare
> W. H. Davies, *Songs of Joy* (1911)

The fight/flight syndrome

First of all let's explain that stress itself is neither harmful nor dangerous – what causes problems is the way we respond to it.

Many tens of thousands of years ago our early ancestors, living in a less complicated prehistoric world, understood little of stress other than that caused by an unexpected confrontation with rather large creatures who had it in mind to snap them up as a tasty snack. So what did our early relations learn to do when confronted with these hungry beasts? They had two options – they could stand and fight or they could turn and run.

For both of these options they needed either extra strength or speed; and so their bodies soon learned that to survive they had to provide the energy for that speed or strength. The heart beat faster, muscles tensed, blood pressure rose, they fought or they ran – and those whose bodies reacted best to their fears survived and lived to fight or run another day. Other changes that they didn't notice also developed – the liver pumped out extra glucose and fats for instant energy, and just in case they were injured in the encounter their blood learned to clot more easily.

And so over the centuries our bodies also learned that when confronted with anything that our minds consider to be a threat to our well-being, we automatically move into the 'fight or flight' mode. Just as it was for our ancestors, so it is for us – our blood pressure rises, our sugar and fat levels increase, our blood becomes 'thicker', our hearts beat faster and we are ready to either fight or run like hell!

But in this modern age it isn't that easy. Our concerns aren't ones that can be solved by fighting or running. The fears that arise in our sophisticated world are more to do with paying the mortgage, insecurity in our workplace or difficulties within our relationships. They are not fears that can easily be appeased by physical action.

Yet our bodies don't know that; they automatically respond to thousands of years of conditioning and at the first sign of anxiety or concern, up goes the blood pressure, faster beats the heart and the

---

Your body under stress

Here's how your body reacts to stress:

- heart rate increases
- blood pressure rises
- blood vessels narrow
- increased blood flow to the muscles
- muscles tense
- blood sugar and fat levels rise
- blood becomes thicker and more likely to clot.

If you have heart disease the increase in your heart rate, together with raised blood pressure, will increase your heart's need for oxygen and may bring on angina. If your blood tends to clot it could also lead to a clot in your artery and trigger a heart attack. Most of these changes are due to an excess production of adrenalin.

whole body becomes poised ready for physical action. But for us there is no physical action – our modern problems don't require it.

For our ancestors the fight or flight lasted only a few minutes; they either survived or they joined the food chain. If they survived they could retire to relax in their cave, their physical changes spent. But we can't solve our modern problems like that – they stay with us day in and day out, week in and week out – and so the fight/flight reaction never switches off.

How can we manage stress?

The first thing to remember is that it's not what happens to us that causes us stress, but rather it's how we react to what has happened. The following suggestions should help you focus on your reactions to situations, rather than the situation itself.

- *Recognize the signs.* Stress is like a large ball rolling down a hill – the further it gets, the more difficult it is to stop it.
- *Identify the cause of your stress.* As the old saying goes – know thine enemy!
- *Try to avoid circumstances that lead to stress.* Remember our ancestors – they very quickly learned that it was wiser to avoid big beasty than come face-to-face with him.
- *Get organized.* It'll help you anticipate and avoid situations in the future that could lead to stress.
- *Remember your priorities.* You know, those important things in life – family and friends; loving and sharing; those quiet moments reading or working in the garden; that favourite hobby.
- *Keep things in proportion.* If you miss a bus, well, there'll always be another one.
- *Don't aim your expectations too high.* Isn't our contentment measured by the difference between our expectations and the reality?
- *Make sure you get sufficient rest.* There's nothing like tiredness to exaggerate our perception of things. Avoid making decisions when you are tired.
- *Improve your communication skills.* It will help others understand your needs and desires and be more in tune with you.
- *Laugh a lot.* It may not be the best medicine in the world but it certainly helps.
- *Take time out.* Our ancestors spent more time relaxing than

running. We must learn to stop and let life's worries flow out of our body and mind.

Where we find stress

Stress comes in many varied guises and we all respond to different situations in different ways. And not all stress stems from negative situations either: the birth of a child, for instance, or going on a holiday, are both joyful events yet each carries with it elements that will give us stress.

Here's a list of situations that at some time or another we may come across in our lives and will have a bearing on our well-being.

death of a loved one	pregnancy
divorce	marriage
marital break-up	marital reconciliation
personal illness	financial problems
loss of a job	retirement
sexual problems	going on holiday
death of a close friend	Christmas
change of job	graduation
selling a house	buying a house
sickness	having an operation

Some pointers on reducing stress

- The most important point of all – *look after yourself*. Eat a healthy diet, take regular exercise and don't let yourself get tired. If you need a nap in the afternoon or early evening – take it.
- *Live in the present.* Too many people spend too much time either regretting the past or worrying about the future.
- *Be optimistic.* Look at your glass as being half-full rather than half-empty.
- Learn the difference between *worrying* about things and being *concerned* about them. Champions win games because they concern themselves with the game, not because they worry about its outcome.
- Try out some of the different *relaxation disciplines* – t'ai chi, meditation, contemplation, prayer or yoga – and take up one that you feel comfortable with. All the ancient civilizations discovered the value of effective relaxation – we should use their wisdom.

Stress-reducing techniques

Do you ever get the feeling when you're very stressed that if only you weren't so stressed you'd have all the time in the world to get all those things done that seem to be building up on you? And how often have you listened to a friend go on about how busy they are and you're screaming inside that if only they stopped talking about it and got on with it there wouldn't be a problem!

A good way to describe this condition is 'overload'. So much to do – so little time. And one of the annoying things about 'overload' is that it's an accumulating condition – like that large stone rolling down a hill, the more momentum it has, the more difficult it is to stop.

One of the ways around this is to learn one of the traditional stress-reducing techniques. The advantage of these is that they are techniques that once learned can be turned to at any time, either in anticipation of stress or to offer relief from it.

Meditation

Meditation has been practised in India and much of Asia for many centuries as a way of achieving spiritual enlightenment. In the 1960s The Beatles 'discovered' Maharishi Mahesh Yogi and brought the practice of meditation to a far wider audience.

Although forms of meditation are practised by various religious orders – both Christian and non-Christian – its popularity in the West has centred on its benefits as a self-help method of stress release.

The practice involves sitting quietly in a comfortable environment for 20–30 minutes focusing attention on a particular thought – maybe an image or sound, or perhaps your breath as you breathe in and out. Whatever you choose, this is called your 'mantra'. Should your attention stray – which in your early days it certainly will – you must gently bring it back to your original focus.

With time you will find it much easier to relax and hold your 'mantra' steady in your mind and you'll soon find yourself letting go of the distractions and anxieties which create stress in your life. It does take time, but the rewards when you have learned how to meditate are rich indeed, for it will help you find a new perspective to your life and perhaps reflect on where your priorities should lie.

For meditation to be effective you should learn it from a trained teacher – then once learned it is a skill you will be able to use for ever.

Yoga

The word yoga comes from the Sanskrit for 'yoke' or 'union'. Its underlying philosophy brings together mind and body, and stresses that both are necessary if we are to enjoy the full benefits of physical exercise.

Yoga is made up of a series of related exercises and postures designed to promote physical, mental and spiritual well-being.

It is interesting to note that just as it was a musical group that brought meditation to the notice of the West, so it was a musician who first made us aware of yoga. In the early 1960s the violinist Sir Yehudi Menuhin's career was threatened by a recurring shoulder problem. After a series of yoga lessons the shoulder improved, and the world was again able to enjoy the master's virtuoso performances.

T'ai-chi ch'uan

The beginnings of t'ai-chi ch'uan can be traced back to China in the eleventh century. A Taoist thinker, considering the nature of the martial arts, observed a largish bird pecking at a snake and was impressed by the way the snake moved slowly and continuously as it evaded the attentions of its attacker. Such movements were studied in relation to the characteristics of other animals and eventually adopted by Taoist monks in their monasteries as a way of integrating body, mind and spirit by combining movement with breathing. Over the years t'ai-chi ch'uan has developed into its modern form, yet many of the movements still reflect its early beginnings – 'riding the tiger', 'resisting the monkey', etc.

Usually known by its shortened name, t'ai chi, meaning wellness, it is a series of slow-moving, dance-like movements which encourage body awareness, balance and confidence.

Dos and don'ts about yoga and t'ai chi

- *Do* take lessons from a qualified teacher and see if you can find one who is specially concerned with stress relaxation.
- *Do* consult your doctor before you begin either discipline.
- *Don't* complete with others in your class – it's not a sport.
- *Do* practise every day.
- *Do* wear loose and comfortable clothing.
- *Don't* practise either yoga or t'ai chi on a full stomach.
- *Do* take a shower before and after exercising as it will help you relax.

Depression

It's quite common for anyone having a heart attack, or having been diagnosed with heart disease, to experience feelings of depression. Unlike stress, depression has an almost reverse effect on us. Rather than wanting to fight or run, we become lethargic, have a sense of helplessness and an inability to move our thoughts or feelings beyond ourselves and our self pity: very normal, very understandable and, fortunately, very quick to pass.

Overcoming depression

- If you, or someone close to you, experience feelings of depression the very first and best thing you should do is talk about it. Share the feelings and fears and the chances are that you'll find the simple act of talking is like a tonic in itself.
- Get exercising. When your body's active it produces natural antidepressant hormones called 'endorphins' and you'll find even a short walk will help to ease the mind. If you keep up the exercising you should soon be back to your normal cheery self.
- Set simple tasks for yourself. Perhaps get one of those model kits and make up a boat, a car or a plane. Or maybe you prefer a not too complicated jigsaw puzzle – whatever. You may find it hard at first but look upon it as a start to feeling better.

If the depression persists have a talk with your doctor – it could be that you'll be put on one of the anti-depression medications.

Never forget – we are body, mind and spirit. *Don't neglect any of these – they are important, interconnected and interdependent.*

Travelling and heart disease

A traveller without knowledge is a bird without wings.

Sa'di, *Gulistan* (1258)

If you have heart disease and your condition is stable, then you should have no worries about travelling. If, however, you have unstable angina, uncontrolled heart failure or serious rhythm disturbances, then you should have these well under control before setting out away from home. We'd also advise you not to fly long distances for about six weeks after heart surgery or heart attack – in fact the airlines may not let you.

Listed below are a few hints that we hope will make your travelling safer and more enjoyable.

- *Drugs* Take sufficient medicine to last you the whole trip. In fact we recommend that you also take a spare set of medicines in case one gets lost. Have one set in your hand luggage, the other packed in your suitcase. Just to be on the safe side, keep a list of the medication you're on with your travel documents.
- *Time zones* If you're changing time zones, talk it over with your doctor to see how it will affect the medication you're on. It's probably best to travel using your home time zone, and then make any changes to your medication time on your arrival. But do get some advice.
- *Heart history* Before you leave, get a letter from your GP or cardiologist with details of your heart history and keep it with you on your trip. If you've had a recent heart attack or surgery, it would be a good idea to also carry a copy of your ECG (electrocardiogram).
- *Anticoagulants* If you are taking warfarin, this will need to be controlled while you're overseas. The measurement for warfarin control is called INR (international normalized ratio), which means that in most countries the result of your test is the same. But do talk with your doctor before you leave and ask for the results of recent tests and the dose of warfarin you've needed to achieve those results. If possible, try to control the warfarin by dosing yourself. You'll need a doctor overseas to refer you to a laboratory, although new finger-prick warfarin tests are now available; but be warned – they are expensive.
- *Airport security* Although pacemakers and post-surgery wires in the chest don't usually trigger the airport security systems, there could be a chance that they might. For this reason it's a good idea to carry a letter saying that you have a pacemaker or that you have had open heart surgery.
- *Insurance* It's best to be open with your travel agent about your heart condition.
- *Luggage* Be careful and selective in what you pack; most passengers take far too many clothes and use only a few. Use

luggage that is easy to move around, preferably with wheels. Always carry your documents, money and other valuable belongings with you in your hand luggage.
- *Avoid rushing* Plan to arrive at the airport early rather than at the last minute – remember traffic is often unpredictable. Avoid carrying heavy suitcases: use trolleys as much as you can, or alternatively use a porter. (You'll be amazed how quickly they can take you to the top of the queue!) Try to avoid tight airline connections – there will always be another plane (and usually, though not always, the airline will put you up in a hotel if you miss a connecting flight).
- *Clothes* Wear comfortable, loose clothes while travelling – it's not a fashion parade. If you feel cold, ask for a blanket – all planes carry them. Find out what the weather is likely to be at your destination, and have appropriate clothing in your hand luggage.
- *Air pressure* Most planes are pressurized and for most of us this doesn't present a problem. However, if you have heart failure or a severe airway disease such as emphysema, bronchitis, etc., you should discuss this with both your doctor and the airline.
- *Meals* Airline food is reasonably harmless, although if you have a heart condition we would advise you to order low-fat, low-salt meals when you're making your reservations. These are generally of a high quality and often tastier than meals provided for other passengers.
- *If you should feel unwell* Don't be shy – tell one of your flight attendants. They are very well trained and equipped for emergencies. They will also know if there is a doctor or nurse on board who can help.
- *Wheelchairs* Most modern airports have long walks to and from the planes and you may well find such a distance difficult. Not to worry – tell somebody at the check-in (or on the plane before you land) that you would like some assistance, and a wheelchair will always be provided. This also usually results in your getting some VIP treatment as well!

DVT (deep vein thrombosis)

Commonly known as *economy class syndrome*.

Long-distance airline travel can cause clots to form in the legs and sometimes these can break off and block the arteries leading to the lungs (pulmonary embolism). This is usually due to a combination of dehydration and lack of movement.

Precautions you can take

- Reduce the length of your flights by planning stopovers whenever possible.
- Wear comfortable shoes and clothes.
- Drink plenty of water.
- A little alcohol with your meal is fine but be careful as alcohol taken in planes can cause dehydration.
- Choose a seat on the aisle and every now and again get up and walk a little.
- Stretch your legs forward as much as you can when resting, as it is bending at the knees and hips that causes the blood to flow less freely.
- Don't cross your legs.

6
Body, mind and spirit

> Man is not the sum of what he has already, but rather the sum of what he does not yet have, of what he could have.
> Jean-Paul Sartre, 'Temporalité' *Situations* (1947–49)

No other part of the human body has played such an important role in our imagination as our heart. From the very earliest days man has linked his emotions, some would say his soul, with his heart.

When we love we 'give our hearts' to the one we love. If it is accepted we can be accused of being 'lighthearted'; if rejected we are 'heartbroken'. If we are brave, it is said that we 'never lose heart' or we have a 'heart of oak', though if we are cowardly we are accused of 'faintheartedness'. We take an oath of allegiance with our 'hand over our heart', making a promise we 'cross our hearts (and hope to die!)'.

And what of the songs we sing – there's poor old Elvis breaking his heart at the Heartbreak Hotel, while careless Tony Bennett leaves his in San Francisco!

With such a long-standing and potent relationship between our lives and our hearts, it shouldn't surprise us to learn that there is a strong link between our minds and the welfare of our physical heart.

The lonely heart

In his latest book, *Love & Survival*, Dr Dean Ornish, Clinical Professor of Medicine at the University of California – best known for his studies in proving there can be reversal of heart disease through changing one's lifestyle – proposes that the real epidemic in modern culture is not only physical heart disease but also emotional and spiritual disease, the contributing factors being loneliness, isolation, alienation and depression. He says,

> I have no intention of diminishing the power of diet and exercise, or, for that matter, of drugs and surgery. There is more scientific evidence now than ever before demonstrating how simple changes in diet and lifestyle may cause significant improvements in health and well being. As important as these are, I have found

that perhaps the most powerful intervention is the healing power of love and intimacy. (Dean Ornish, MD: *Love & Survival: 8 Pathways to Intimacy and Health*, HarperCollins, 1998)

The language of the heart, it seems, carries a truth we are only now beginning to understand.

Sharing your feelings

From the moment we're born and suckled at our mother's breast we are inextricably connected to other people. Our lives become part and parcel of those of others; we're part of a family, we go to nursery and school with other young people, we play sports in teams, we get a job as part of a workforce; throughout our lives we make strong friendships. We are each and every one of us part of each other. As John Donne said some 400 years ago – not one of us is an island.

So why is it that when confronted with heart disease many of us – particularly men – tend to hide it away inside ourselves and not want to share how we feel with even those closest to them? Most probably it's denial – it's not easy confronting our own mortality. And sure, there'll be some frustration and anger mixed up in there as well.

However, whatever the cause, it is not a very wise thing to harbour it inside you. Numerous studies have shown that self-disclosure – talking about your feelings – certainly helps you confront and manage the cause of your concern.

So do share your feelings with your loved ones, because in that act alone you will have taken a huge step on your road to recovery, and all those things that seem like chores – like diet, exercise and stress – you'll find just fall into place.

Sexual relationships

Let's first of all get rid of a couple of long-held myths; firstly the myth that after a heart attack you'll have to give up on sex – fortunately, not so at all! The second myth is that after a heart attack you won't be interested in sex – well, yes, true for the first week or so, but then it will very quickly all get back to normal.

Just like any major crisis in one's life, the worry and concern that heart disease engenders will naturally dim sexual desires, and as we well know, any form of mental stress will affect not only our arousal but also our physical performance.

BODY, MIND AND SPIRIT

So if you have heart disease or you've had a heart attack or perhaps surgery, here are a few things you should keep in mind:

- Having sex presents no danger whatsoever, though for six to eight weeks after surgery you should avoid putting weight or pressure on the chest.
- Anxiety over sexual performance is quite normal among couples where one has a heart condition.
- Remember, even though you may be the one with the heart condition, your partner is also going through much the same mental strain as you are.
- Talk openly with each other – a shared problem becomes half a problem.
- While impromptu sex can be exciting, it may be preferable if in the early days you plan it for when you are rested and can be comfortable.
- Medication can interfere with both sexual arousal and performance, and you should talk these matters over with your doctor.
- The demands on your heart when having sex are much the same as going for a brisk walk, washing the car or climbing a couple of flights of stairs.

There are many excellent books on all aspects of sexual relationships and we would strongly recommend you pop down to your local bookshop or library – walking of course! – and choose one that meets your needs.

Viagra

In recent years Viagra (sildenafil) has been hailed as a wonder drug which, its makers claim, can bring joy and excitement back into the lives of impotent men. Apparently, if you're fit, well and healthy this is no idle boast.

However, if you are on nitrates or have any form of heart disease or heart condition, have had a heart attack, have low blood pressure, suffer angina or are on medication of any sort, you should most probably not take Viagra.

Fortunately, in the UK Viagra is a prescription medicine and you can only obtain it with your doctor's approval.

Do not even think about taking it without your doctor's consent – it could well kill you.

(See Appendix B – Suggested reading, p. 103.)

BODY, MIND AND SPIRIT

The power of the mind

The frustrating thing about having a mind of our own is that we sometimes completely forget we have one, and the older we get the more we tend to ignore it. Somehow we seem to overlook the fact that we have the ability to harness this great friend and ally and let it help us take control of our attitudes and emotions.

If we allow the problems of life to constantly dominate our thinking, then those negative thoughts will feed into our subconscious and act as confirmation of our negativity. However, if we work together with our mind and feed it thoughts of well-being, even if we don't feel all that well, then the power of the mind will work towards making those positive thoughts a reality.

Beyond positive thinking

If you wake up one morning and for some perverse reason you tell yourself you're going to be miserable all day, and you keep repeating it to your family and friends, it's not difficult to imagine that by about lunchtime you are going to be a very unhappy person indeed!

The secret is in knowing and believing that there is a powerful link between our mind and our body, and that we have the power to influence and strengthen that link so that our subconscious mind will make our thoughts a reality. By working together with this tremendous positive force it is possible to change our reality. It needs practice – and practice, and more practice! – but it is possible. It's well worth a try.

Here are a few suggestions to get you on your way:

- Think of things as right, good and happy rather than wrong, bad and sad.
- Be creative in your thinking – dismiss negative thoughts from your mind and replace them with positive ones.
- Repeat positive thoughts to yourself throughout the day. Write them down.
- If you daydream make sure the dreams are happy ones. Who dreams of losing the lottery!
- Be positive in your thinking – the bottle should be half-full rather than half-empty.
- Don't worry about things you have no control over.

Get it right and you'll discover that even unexpected dark clouds can have quite wonderful silver linings.

The strength of the spirit

In learning to control our mind and encourage it towards steadily improving our health through positive thoughts and feeling, we call on that intangible part of us that is the very fundamental, emotional and activating principle of our being – our 'spirit'.

Deep inside us, under layers of conditioning, is this force of life that animates our bodies and governs our beliefs and our behaviour. Some express this spirit in the celebration of their religion, promoting times of quiet, meditation and prayer. For others, their spirituality is in the celebration of nature – flowers, trees, the waters of rivers, the sounds of birds and the cool feel of the breeze. The great musicians, writers, poets and painters found their spiritual satisfaction in expressing their art. And, if one is cynical, in recent times the celebration of spirit seems to be in the pursuit of 'things'.

However we choose to acknowledge this force of life, this spirit, it is part of our being and has a strong influence on our ability to positively influence our minds and our lives. We should learn of it and understand it, for in so doing we will positively affect our minds, which in turn will positively affect our bodies; so that all in all we will be much richer. Our spirit links us to a power far greater than any power we possess ourselves and, if we neglect it, we will be infinitely the poorer.

A final word

Here is a final word from actor Ralph Fiennes. When asked in an interview, 'Don't fame and success isolate you from what you were before, and from those you loved?' He replied:

'Success? Well, I don't know quite what you mean by success. Material success? Worldly success? Personal, emotional success? The people I consider successful are so because of how they handle their responsibilities to other people, how they approach the future, people who have a full sense of the value of their life and what they want to do with it.

'I call people "successful" not because they have money or their business is doing well, but because as human beings, they have a fully developed sense of being alive and engaged in a life-time task

Fact or fiction?

Elsewhere in this book we've talked about the important role our heart plays in our imagination and how we've linked it to our emotions. It has become central to almost everything we do – we fall in love with our heart, our heroes are strong-hearted, and our villains have no heart at all.

Is it any surprise then to learn that there are many myths that have grown over the years concerning our hearts and that those myths have crossed over to the things that can go wrong with it?

So let's have a look at the five most common of these fanciful myths.

- *Heart disease is an old man's disease.* Not true. Though an awful lot of old men develop heart disease it is in fact a disease that more often than not has its beginnings in adolescence and progressively develops throughout our lives. If it is diagnosed early enough there's much we can do to prevent it raising its ugly head. (See Beating the odds, p. 45.)
- *Women are unlikely to get heart disease.* Not true. The sad fact is that women are more likely to die of heart disease than that which scares them most – breast cancer. (See Men's hearts, women's hearts, p. 4.)
- *Once you have heart disease – well, that's it!* Not true. Every year, as we learn more about heart disease that old myth is shown for what it is – a myth. Over the last decade we've learned that with the right diet, a reasonable amount of exercise and a little help from modern medication, we can not only hold the disease in check, but in many cases actually reverse it. (See Beating the odds, p. 45.)
- *After a heart attack you may as well give up.* Not true. Modern rehabilitation techniques mean that after a heart attack or other major cardiac event you can recover to enjoy a full and meaningful life. (See Beating the odds, p. 45.)
- *When you exercise your heart will only benefit if you sweat a lot.* Not true. If you want to run in the Olympics, OK you follow the 'no pain – no gain' philosophy and you could win a medal. But if all you want to do is to lower the risk of heart disease, then all you really need is to 'accumulate' about 30 minutes of moderate exercise on as many days as you can. (See Keeping the body moving, p. 70.)

of collaboration with other human beings – their mothers and fathers, their family, their friends, their loved ones, the friends who are dying, the friends who are being born.

'Success?' he repeated emphatically. 'Don't you know it is all about being able to extend love to people? Not in a big, capital-letter sense, but in the everyday, little-by-little, task-by-task, gesture-by-gesture, word-by-word.'

7
Dietary supplements

Sup+ple-ment: 1. n. an addition designed to complete, make up for a deficiency; 2. v. to provide a supplement to, in order to remedy a deficiency.

The manufacture and supply of dietary supplements is now a multibillion-dollar business throughout the Western world. Embraced by an ageing baby-boomer generation, a whole variety of supplements are readily available not only in pharmacies and health shops, but also in an ever-growing number of supermarkets.

However, many dietary and medical professionals are not convinced that we should be putting such a strong emphasis on looking to supplements to meet our dietary needs.

To supplement or not to supplement?

Let's first of all look at three important facts:

Fact 1 To work properly our body's cells need to get all the nutrients they were designed to receive.
Fact 2 We can only get these nutrients from ingesting them in the food we eat.
Fact 3 Our bodies will survive with lesser quantities of these nutrients, but may be more prone to diseases.

What the pro-vitamin school of thought argues is as follows:

- That modern farming depletes the soil of many of the nutrients and micronutrients we need.
- Because fewer nutrients are added to the soil, more sprays, often toxic, are used. Antioxidants protect against the resulting free radical damage. (See Antioxidants, p. 65.)
- Many of our fruit and vegetables are picked early, before all their nutrient value has been created.
- We store, freeze, process and then reheat much of our food and in doing so we destroy many of the nutrients.

Given these as truths, it seems that supplementing our diet isn't a bad thing after all.

But then in comes the anti-supplement lobby: 'Where is your evidence?' they ask. 'Can you give us scientific proof that taking supplements will actually benefit you?' Unfortunately, it is unlikely that this will ever be proven one way or the other for a number of reasons.

- Trials cost huge amounts of money and as vitamins and natural substances cannot be patented it is unlikely that anyone will fund a trial relating to an unprotected product.
- Furthermore, most supplements work in combinations – so a trial of just one supplement is unlikely to give any meaningful results. For example, vitamin E needs vitamin C, selenium and coenzyme Q10 to work best, so if a trial were to be positive, how would we know which supplement caused the result?
- As supplements are really just 'good complete food' the diet of people in the trial may affect the results. (For example, a recent trial of vitamin E in Mediterranean people did not show any benefit from taking vitamin E supplements. But Mediterranean food itself has a high vitamin E content – so those not on vitamin E tablets were still getting vitamin E.)

So where does all this leave our poor patient who just wants to do what's best for the body? It seems no one can definitively prove that supplements are good for you, and yet no one can say they aren't. It's a matter for the individual and the only advice we can offer is that if you truly believe supplementing your diet will be beneficial, then the chances are it will be.

However, may we suggest that before making any decision about supplements you talk it over with your doctor.

A word of warning – taking supplements doesn't let you off the hook from eating properly; you must still keep to a healthy diet.

The supplements that may help your heart

Antioxidants

When the cholesterol in the plaque in our arteries becomes oxidized, it can rupture and cause a heart attack. Antioxidants such as vitamins E, C and A, selenium and coenzyme Q10 can help prevent this. (See We are what we eat, p. 54.)

DIETARY SUPPLEMENTS

Homocysteine-reducing vitamins

High levels of homocysteine in the blood contribute to the narrowing of arteries. Recent studies have shown that vitamins B6, B12 and folic acid can control this. (See Blood cholesterol, p. 25.)

Niacin (nicotinic acid; a B complex vitamin)

Niacin lowers levels of bad cholesterol and raises that of the good. It is also one of the few drugs that can lower the bad lipoprotein (a) cholesterol. Unfortunately it can cause quite unpleasant flushing, although new 'no flush' preparations are now available and niacin may soon become a front-line cholesterol-lowering drug.

Selenium

Selenium works together with vitamin E as an antioxidant.

Coenzyme Q10

An essential nutrient in every cell of our body, coenzyme Q10 (also known as ubiquinone) is required to produce energy. Although its use is not supported by the conventional medical community there are a number of studies showing it may have benefits for heart failure and heart rhythm disorders. In conjunction with vitamin E it is a powerful antioxidant.

Fish oils

People in communities which have a high level of fish in their diet tend to have a low incidence of heart disease. The omega-3 oils in fish – also found in flaxseed (linseed) oil – have beneficial effects on blood clotting, stabilizing artery walls and heart rhythms. (See We are what we eat, p. 54.)

Magnesium

Magnesium is needed by many of our cells, including those in our heart. People given intravenous magnesium after a heart attack recover better and have fewer complications, suggesting that it may be lacking in our cells. It is thought that it may also stabilize some heart rhythm disorders. It also helps relax our muscles, thus helping us get a good night's sleep. (See We are what we eat, p. 54.)

Garlic

Garlic has long been seen as being good for the health, and people living in countries in which garlic is widely eaten have lower rates of heart disease – but whether it's the garlic or other factors still remains to be proven. (See We are what we eat, p. 54.)

Appendix A
The drugs we take

We've come a long way since the days when doctors roamed the land with little bottles full of leeches that they used to cure our ills. And thank goodness for that! Now, in our wonderful modern world it's little bottles of coloured pills that doctors turn to to fight our maladies.

So let's have a look at these little coloured tablets that so many of us rely on. The drugs are listed by their generic names rather than their brand names. Both names should always be on the label of any prescribed drug.

Common medications for various heart conditions

Medication for high blood pressure
Diuretics
Beta-blockers
ACE inhibitors
Calcium-channel blockers
Alpha-blockers

Medication for high cholesterol
Statins
Fibrates
Niacin
Bile-acid binders

Medication for coronary artery disease
Beta-blockers
Aspirin
Calcium-channel blockers
Nitrates
Calcium antagonists
ACE inhibitors

Medication for heart failure
ACE inhibitors
Digoxin
Diuretics

Nitrates
Beta-blockers

Details of the more commonly prescribed medication

ACE (angiotensin-converting enzyme) inhibitors

What they do
They lower blood pressure and improve the circulation.

How they do it
Our kidneys release a hormone (angiotensin) that causes small arteries to contract, thus raising blood pressure. ACE inhibitors block this hormone and thereby lower blood pressure.

Possible side-effects
Dry cough, headache, metallic taste, dizziness (if the blood pressure gets too low).

Generic name
Captopril
Enalapril
Lisinopril
Quinapril
Cilazopril

Alpha-blockers

What they do
They lower blood pressure.

How they do it
They relax small blood vessels.

Possible side-effects
Common side-effects are tiredness, headache, dizziness (especially when first started).

Generic name
Doxazosin
Prazosin
Terazosin

Antiarrhythmics

What they do
They stabilize heart rhythm disorders.

How they do it
Irregular heartbeats are usually caused by an upset in the electrical system which keeps the heart ticking over. Antiarrhythmics attempt to stabilize this – not always successfully.

Remember Most palpitations and irregular beating are quite benign and worry you more than your doctor. Make sure your symptoms really need treating before starting on some of these powerful medicines. Also look at relaxation and dietary approaches (see Coping with stress, p. 75 and Dietary supplements – magnesium, p. 94).

There are a large number of antiarrhythmic drugs, for different rhythms and symptoms. The most commonly used ones are:

Beta-blockers
Calcium-channel blockers
Amiodarone
Flecainide

Possible side-effects
These drugs have a number of side-effects specific to each. You should ask your doctor about these before starting them.

Anticoagulants

What they do
They reduce the blood's tendency to clot and lower the risk of emboli and stroke for people with atrial fibrillation, artificial heart valves and leg thrombosis.

How they do it
They interfere with the production of blood-clotting factors.

Possible side-effects
Common: bleeding.

If you are taking anticoagulants you should mention this to your dentist or doctor before dental procedures or surgery.

Generic name
Warfarin

Interaction with food and drugs
There are some foods that can affect the action of warfarin. You don't need to avoid these foods, but try to eat reasonably consistent

amounts so the effect on the INR (international normalized ratio) will be uniform.

The following foods will *reduce* the effects of warfarin: avocado, broccoli, Brussels sprouts, raw cabbage, chick-peas, green beans, green tea, liver, lettuce, raw spinach.

Some drugs will also affect warfarin action. These will *reduce* its effect: barbiturates, carbamazepine, chlordiazepoxide, colestyramine, griseofulvin, oral contraceptives, rifampicin, sucralfate, vitamin K.

These will *increase* its effect: amiodarone, aspirin, anabolic steroids, cimetidine, ciprofloxacin, clofibrate, danazol, disulfiram, erythromycin, imidazole, isoniazid, metronidazole, non-steroidal anti-inflammatory drugs (NSAIDs), proton pump inhibitors, propranolol, quinidine, statins, thyroxine, tricyclic antidepressants, verapamil.

Check this list before starting any new drug, and if it is on the list you'll need more blood tests to check your INR.

Aspirin
What it does
In low doses it changes the platelets – the clotting cells in the blood – and makes them less sticky. This reduces clotting and thrombosis – and reduces the incidence and severity of heart attacks.

Possible side-effects
Aspirin can irritate the stomach, cause increased bleeding, and in some people make their asthma worse.

Generic name
Aspirin

Beta-blockers
What they do
They reduce the blood pressure and slow and stabilize the heartbeat.

How they do it
They block the action of excess adrenalin, which enables the heart to beat more slowly, thus allowing the heart muscle to use less oxygen, while also lowering blood pressure.

Possible side-effects
Common: aggravates asthma and some lung disorders, impotence, tiredness, heightened dreams, cold fingers and toes. Less common: depression.

Generic name
Atenolol
Metoprolol
Celiprilol
Sotolol
Pindolol
Nadolol
Propranolol
Timolol
Oxprenolol
Labetolol

Note: *If you have asthma you should not take beta-blockers.*

Calcium-channel blockers
What they do
They lower blood pressure and control angina.

How they do it
They open up blood vessels and slow the heart rate.

Possible side-effects
Common: headaches, swelling of the ankles, constipation, nausea.

Note Some calcium-channel blockers (verapamil and diliazem) work in a similar way to beta-blockers, *and the two groups should only be used together with caution.*

Generic name
Verapamil
Diltiazem
Nifedipine
Amlodipine
Felodipine
Isradipine
Nisoldipine
Lacidipine
Lercanidipine

Cholesterol-lowering drugs – statins, niacin and fibrates
1 Statins
What they do
They lower cholesterol.

How they do it
They reduce the cholesterol that is produced by the liver.

Possible side-effects
Common: liver function problems, upset stomach.
Rare (but very important): muscle aching. If this happens, stop the drug and tell your doctor.

Generic name
Atorvastatin
Fluvastatin
Lovastatin
Pravastatin
Simvastatin

2 Niacin

(See Dietary supplements, p. 92.)

What it does
It lowers cholesterol.

How it does it
Niacin is a B-complex vitamin, B3, that restricts the body's production of bad cholesterol (LDL) and raises the good HDL.

Possible side-effects
Common: flushing, itching, headaches. Some 'no flush' brands are now on the market.

3 Fibrates

How they work
They lower levels of triglycerides by blocking their production in the liver; fibrates also raise the good HDL.

Possible side-effects
Most common: nausea, upset stomach, stomach pains, vomiting, gas.
Less common: headache, rash, itching, dizziness.

Generic name
Bezafibrate
Gemfibrozil
Clofibrate

Ciprofibrate
Fenofibrate

Diuretics

What they do
They lower blood pressure, and in cases of congestive heart failure they reduce swelling and the accumulation of fluid.

How they do it
High blood-sodium levels elevate blood pressure and cause water retention. Diuretics induce the kidneys to remove sodium.

Possible side-effects
Lower potassium levels with most diuretics (which can cause nausea and tiredness), impotence, cramps, dizziness.

Thiazide diuretics
Generic name
Clorothiazide
Cyclopenthiazide
Bendrofluazide

Loop diuretics
Generic name
Frusemide
Bumetanide

Potassium-sparing diuretics
Generic name
Amiloride
Spironolactone
Triamterene

Nitrates

What they do
They help to prevent and treat angina.

How they do it
Nitrates dilate blood vessels, thus decreasing the heart's workload and increasing the blood flow through partly blocked coronary arteries, and open collateral vessels.

Possible side-effects
Common: headaches, flushing, increased pulse, sweating, faintness when standing.

Note If you're on nitrates you should not take the anti-impotence medication Viagra (see Viagra, p. 87).

Generic name
Isosorbide mononitrate
Isosorbide dinitrate
Glyceryl trinitrate

Vasodilators

What they do
They lower blood pressure.

How they do it
They dilate blood vessels. (Vasodilators are often used in conjunction with other blood pressure-lowering drugs such as diuretics and beta-blockers.)

Possible side-effects
Common: headache, increased heart rate, flushing.

Note If you have coronary artery disease, vasodilators if given alone may aggravate angina symptoms.

Generic name
Hydralazine
Minoxidil

Note If you're taking any of the vasodilators you may feel dizzy when standing after being in a sitting or lying position. This is particularly noticeable if you stand up very quickly; to avoid this, make sure you keep your movement slow. Of itself, it is not a matter for concern, the cause being no more than a sudden drop in your blood pressure.

Appendix B
Suggested reading

The following is a list of books we recommend if you're looking for more information on specific issues. They aren't the only books that cover these subject matters and for a more comprehensive selection we recommend that you go to your local bookshop or library – walking of course! – and see if there is something that better meets your needs.

General
Topol, Eric J. MD (ed.), *Cleveland Clinic Heart Book*, Hyperion Press, 2000.

Gersh, Bernard J. MD (ed.), *Mayo Clinic Heart Book*, William Morrow Press, 1993.

Antioxidants
Youngson, Dr Robert, *Antioxidants*, Sheldon Press, 1998.

Cholesterol
Povey, Robert, *How to Keep Your Cholesterol in Check*, Sheldon Press, 1997.

Food/cookery
Polunin, Miriam, *Healing Foods*, Dorling Kindersley, 1997.

High blood pressure
Sheps, Sheldon G. MD (ed.), *The Mayo Clinic on High Blood Pressure*, The Mayo Clinic, 1999.

Mind and development
Covey, Stephen and Merrill, Roger, *First Things First*, Prentice Hall, 1996.

Sexual problems
Bonnard, Marc MD, *The Viagra Alternative*, Healing Arts Press, 1999.

Stress
Powell, Dr Trevor, *Stress Free Living*, Dorling Kindersley, 1997.

SUGGESTED READING

Stroke
Swaffield, Laura, *Stroke: The Complete Guide to Recovery and Rehabilitation*, Thorsons Publishing, 1996.
Smith, Dr Tom, *Coping with Strokes*, Sheldon Press, 2000.

Appendix C
Useful addresses

The British Heart Foundation
14 Fitzhardinge Street
London W1H 6DH
Tel: 020 7935 0185
Website: bhf.org.uk
Email: internet@bhf.org.uk

St John Ambulance
27 St John's Lane
London EC1M 4BU
Tel: 08700 104950
Website: sja.org.uk

Diabetes UK
10 Parkway
London NW1 7AA
Tel: 020 7424 1000
Website: diabetes.org.uk
Email: info@diabetes.org.uk

BHF Centre of Physical Activity and Health
Loughborough University
Ashby Road
Loughborough
Leicestershire LE11 3TU
Tel: 01509 223259
Website: bhfactive.org.uk

Walking the Way to Health
Countryside Agency
John Dower House
Crescent Place
Cheltenham GL50 3RA
Tel: 01242 533258
Website: whi.org.uk

USEFUL ADDRESSES

QUIT
(for help in giving up smoking)
Ground Floor
211 Old Street
London EC1V 9NR
Quitline: 0800 002200
Website: quit.org.uk

Action on Smoking and Health
102 Clifton Street
London EC2A 4HW
Tel: 020 7739 5902

NHS Smoking Helpline
0800 169 0169

The Stroke Association
Stroke House
Whitecross Street
London EC1Y 8JJ
Helpline: 0845 303 3100
Website: stroke.org.uk

Glossary

Angiogram A test giving a picture of blood flow through your heart and arteries.
Angioplasty A means of unblocking narrow or blocked arteries with a small balloon.
Arteries The vessels that carry blood away from the heart to all the body's tissues.
Arteriosclerosis A posh way of saying 'narrowing of the arteries'.
Atherosclerosis Another posh way of saying 'narrowing of the arteries'.
Beta-blockers A common drug, prescribed for a number of heart conditions, which blocks the effects of adrenalin.
Cardiovascular The heart and all the blood vessels.
Carotid artery The vessel that supplies the brain with oxygen-rich blood.
Cholesterol The main ingredient of the plaque that causes blocking of the arteries.
Congenital Something that's there when we're born.
Coronary arteries The vessels that carry blood to our heart muscle.
Defibrillator A machine that can restore normal heart rhythm with an electrical shock.
ECG Electrocardiogram: a diagnostic instrument that records how the heart is functioning.
Embolus (plural: emboli) A travelling blood clot.
HDL (high density lipoprotein) cholesterol Good cholesterol.
Hypertension The technical name for high blood pressure.
Hypotension The technical name for low blood pressure.
Ischaemia Where there is reduced blood flow to tissues due to narrowed or blocked arteries.
LDL (low density lipoprotein) cholesterol Bad cholesterol.
Lipids Fats in the blood.
Murmur An abnormal heart noise heard with a stethoscope, usually caused by a valve problem.
Myocardial infarction The technical name for a heart attack.
Myocardium The heart muscle.
Occlusion A blockage – usually in an artery.
Oedema Abnormal swelling due to excess fluid.

GLOSSARY

Pacemaker A small device implanted under the skin which regulates irregular heart rhythms.
Palpitations The sensation of rapid or missed heartbeats.
Plaque The sticky deposit that forms on the inner lining of blood vessels that causes thickening and blockage.
Pulse rate The number of heartbeats per minute.
Re-stenosis The further narrowing of an artery that has been widened by angioplasty or other cardiac procedure.
Stenosis Another way of saying that a blood vessel is narrowed.
Stent An expanding wire-mesh tube used to hold open a narrowed artery after angioplasty.
Thrombus A blood clot.

Index

ACE inhibitors, 9, 96
alcohol, 9, 27, 64–5
alpha-blockers, 96
aneurysm, 10
angina pectoris, 7, 15, 48, 73, 75, 76, 82, 101
  medications for, 7, 99, 101
angiography, 35–6
angioplasty, 38–9
antiarrhythmics, 97
anticoagulants, 42, 82, 97–8
antioxidants, 57, 64, 65, 92, 93
aqua jogging, 74, 75
arrhythmias, 12–14
arterial embolism, 10–11
arteries, 2 – *see also* coronary artery disease; stroke
aspirin, 38, 98
atherosclerosis – *see* coronary artery disease
atrial arrhythmias, 13
atrial septal defect, 12

beans, 60
beta-blockers, 7, 74, 78–9
biscuits, 68
blood pressure, 3–4 – *see also* hypertension
blood tests, 32
bradycardia, 14
bread, 68
breathlessness, 114
British Heart Foundation, 22

calcium, 62
calcium-channel blockers, 7, 74, 99
calcium scoring, 49
capillaries, 2
carbohydrates, 56, 57–60
cardiac arrest, 19, 21
cardiomyopathy, 10

cerebral embolism, haemorrhage or thrombosis, 16
chest pains, 6, 113
cholesterol, 25–7, 28, 29, 61, 66, 67, 71, 93–4
cholesterol-lowering drugs, 95, 99–100
coarctation of the aorta, 12
coenzyme Q10, 93, 94
collapse, sudden, 113–14
congenital heart disease, 11–12
congestive heart failure, 8
coronary artery bypass graft surgery, 39–41, 43
coronary artery disease, 5–7, 25
  medication for, 7, 95
coronary care unit, 21
'couch potato' syndrome, 5, 28, 74
counselling, 47
CPR (cardiopulmonary resuscitation), 20, 22, 114
CT or CAT scan (computerized tomography), 35

dairy products, 60, 66–7
defibrillation, 20, 23
depression, 41, 81, 85
diabetes, 17–18, 24, 68
diagnostic tests, 31–7
diet, 25, 27, 45–6, 51–2, 54–70
dietary supplements, 92–4
digitalis, 9
diuretics, 9, 74, 101
dizziness, 114
drugs, 37–8, 82, 95–102 *see also* specific drugs, e.g. beta-blockers
DVT (deep vein thrombosis), 84

eating out, 70
ECG (electrocardiogram), 33
echocardiography, 35
economy class syndrome, 84
ectopic beats, 13
eggs, 60, 67

109

INDEX

electrical (rhythm) problems, 12–15, 18, 82, 94
embolism
 arterial, 10
 cerebral, 16
emergency guidelines, 112–14
endocarditis, infective, 16
exercise, 9, 27, 28, 46, 47, 52, 70–5, 80, 81, 90

family history, risk of heart disease, 5, 24
family, role of, 49–51
fats, 56, 65–6
feelings, talking about, 23, 41, 81, 86
fibrates, 100
fibrillation, 13–14, 18, 20
fight/flight syndrome, 75–6
fish, 61
fish oils, 94
flavonoids, 59, 64, 65
flaxseed, 61, 94
fluids, 64–5
folic acid, 26, 64
free radicals, 59, 65, 92
fruit, 58

garlic, 59, 94
grains, 59

heart attack, 18–21, 48, 76, 112–13
heart disease – *see also* prevention; risk factors; and specific diseases, e.g. angina
 men and, 4, 18, 24, 29
 myths about, 90
 statistics, ix
 women and, 4, 18, 24, 29, 90
heart block, 14
heart failure, 7, 9, 15, 18, 83
 medication for, 9
 surgery for, 43
heart rate, evaluating, 73
heart, role of, 1
heart transplant, 43
Holter monitoring, 33
homocysteine, 26, 94
hypertension, 9, 27, 71, 73
 medication for, 95, 99, 102

infective endocarditis, 16
ischaemic heart disease – *see* coronary artery disease

'let's get healthy' plan, 46
lifestyle change, 7, 8, 20, 45–6, 49–53, 85–6 – *see also* diet; exercise
liquids, 64–5
love, 85–6, 90–1

magnesium, 62, 94
meat, 60, 66
medication, 37–8, 82, 95–102 – *see also* specific drugs, e.g. beta-blockers
meditation, 79
Mediterranean diet, 57–8
men and heart disease, 4, 18, 24, 29
mind, power of, 88–9
minerals, 56, 62–3
mitral valve prolapse, 15
myocardial infarction, 18–20
myocarditis, 10

niacin, 94, 100
nitrates, 7, 101–2

olive oil, 58, 66, 67, 68
omega-3 fatty acids, 56, 61, 94
organ donation, 44

pacemakers, 14–15, 82
palpitations, 15
patent ductus arteriosus, 12
percutaneous balloon valvuloplasty, 43
physical examination, 31–2
plaque, 5
potassium, 62
prevention, 49 – *see also* diet; exercise
proteins, 56, 60–1
pulmonary oedema, 8
pulmonary stenosis, 12

race, and heart disease, 24
recovery, 21, 40–1, 45–6 – *see also* lifestyle change
regurgitation, valve, 15
rehabilitation, 47–8
rhythm disorders, 12–15, 82, 94
risk factors, ix, 5, 8–9, 25–30

INDEX

St John Ambulance, 22
salt, 9, 27, 63, 67
selenium, 94
sexual relationships, 86–7
sildenafil, 87
sinus node, 12, 14
smoking, xii, 27, 28–30, 46, 52
sodium, 9, 63, 67
soy foods, 61–2
spirituality, 89
statistics, ix
stenosis
 aortic or mitral valve, 15
 pulmonary, 12
stents, 39
stethoscope, 32
stress, 27, 28, 46, 71, 75–80
stress test, 34
stroke, 16–17
sudden cardiac death (cardiac arrest), 21–3
sugar, 68–9
surgery, 39–44, 48
systolic pressure, 3–4

tachycardia, 13–14, 18
t'ai chi, 75, 78, 80
tests, diagnostic, 31–7
thallium stress test, 34
thrombosis
 cerebral, 16
 deep vein, 84
TIAs (transient ischaemic attacks), 16–17

trans-fatty acids, 68
travelling, and heart disease, 81–4
triglycerides, 68, 71, 100

ultrasound, 35
unstable angina, 7

valve problems, 15
 surgery for, 42–3
vasodilators, 7, 102
vegetables, 57
veins, 2
ventricular arrhythmias, 13–14
ventricular septal defect, 12
Viagra, 87, 102
vitamins, 26, 56, 63–4, 92–4
vitamin A, 63
vitamin B, 26, 56, 57, 59, 61, 63–4, 94
vitamin C, 56, 57, 58, 64, 93
vitamin E, 56, 57, 59, 64, 66, 93, 94

walking, 72, 73, 74
warfarin, 42, 82, 97
weight, 27, 68, 71
women and heart disease, 4, 18, 24, 29, 90

x-rays, 33

yoga, 75, 78, 80

At times of crisis

What to do in an emergency or when you don't feel well

This is a quick reference for you and your family in case some unexpected problem arises.

Telephone numbers

Keep important emergency numbers where you can quickly lay your hands on them – preferably near your telephone.

Ambulance / Fire / Police – 999

Other numbers you should have are:

- Your GP
- Emergency medical services
- Local hospital
- Local pharmacy

Warning signs of a heart attack

The classic signs that you are having, or are about to have, a heart attack are not easy to ignore. Whether the symptoms come on suddenly or are a growing, nagging discomfort – do not hesitate – *call an ambulance immediately*. The signs are:

- a strong persistent pressure across the chest, as if an elephant were sitting on it
- pain radiating to your shoulders, back, neck and down your arm or lower jaw
- a burning sensation in the upper abdomen
- shortness of breath, nausea, sweating
- anxiety and fatigue.

AT TIMES OF CRISIS

What to do if you think you're having a heart attack
- Stay as calm as you can.
- Call 999, ask for the ambulance service, and tell them you have chest pain. If you're not up to it get someone else to make the call for you.
- Try to be clear in telling the operator what's wrong and where you are.
- Sit comfortably, loosen your clothing, try to relax and breathe deeply and slowly.
- If you use glyceryl trinitrate tablets or spray, take one or use it and repeat every five minutes.
- If possible chew and swallow an aspirin.

DO NOT!

- Be embarrassed in case it's only heartburn.
- Wait to see if the pain goes away.
- Be concerned about putting anyone out.
- Think you're too young to have a heart attack.
- Try and drive yourself to the hospital.

Remember ...
The sooner you get assistance, the less chance there is of any damage being done. The ambulance staff are proud of what they do and would rather arrive to deal with a false alarm than a dead or dying body.

Chest pains

If you develop persistent chest pains, stop doing the activity that is causing them and sit down somewhere warm. If the pain doesn't go straight away, use your glyceryl trinitrate spray or tablets, taking whatever amount you normally use. (Glyceryl trinitrate works best when you're sitting; if you remain standing the effect can be too strong and you may faint. If you're lying down flat the effect is significantly reduced and you may not get its full benefit.)

Sudden collapse

If somebody feels faint and then collapses the important thing is to keep them lying flat. Check that they are breathing, and have a pulse (feel at either the wrist or neck). If there is neither pulse nor respiration, call the emergency number (999). Then, if you know how, commence CPR. It is best for the person to lie flat, and if they are unconscious it is better if they are rolled onto their side to keep the airway open.

Breathlessness

Breathlessness can sometimes be due to heart failure, and occasionally it may wake you from sleep at night. If this happens it is important you mention it to your doctor. Should you develop breathlessness, stop what you're doing and sit still – sitting is much better than lying down – although do whatever you feel is the most comfortable. Glyceryl trinitrate can often help breathlessness and you can use this every five minutes for three to five doses. If the breathlessness persists, call emergency services.

Dizziness

Some cardiac conditions – and many drugs – can cause your blood pressure to fall when you stand up suddenly. This is quite normal, so don't be worried about it. The best way to overcome it is to get up gradually, and if you've been lying down, sit on the side of the bed for a few seconds before getting up fully and walking away. If you do get dizzy the best thing to do is to lie down for a while. Some people may suggest that you should sit in a chair and put your head between your knees – *don't!* This must be one of the most efficient ways of causing somebody to faint, and should be avoided at all costs. If you feel faint, lie down flat on your back, and preferably with your legs raised above the height of your chest – this allows maximum blood to return to the heart and chest, which is what your body is calling out for.

Palpitations

If you feel your heart racing it is best to sit or lie down for a while – whichever you find most comfortable – and breathe quietly and relax. If the palpitations persist or are causing other symptoms, call the emergency services.